Praise for DON'T TAKE DIET PERSON: From those who have n done the program.

MW00948836

Dr. Alok Kalia, a physician-scientist, has combined his intimate knowledge of medicine, biology and physiology with his personal experience in weight management to produce a book that is immensely practical and scientifically balanced.

Ajit Varki, MD
Distinguished Professor of Medicine and Cellular & Molecular Medicine
Co-Director, Center for Academic Research and Training in Anthropogeny
Co-Director, Glycobiology Research and Training Center
University of California, San Diego

Doctor Alok shows you how to break the cycle of food addiction.

Liz Goodgold—Speaker, Author, Coach (RedfireBranding.com)

After being on Doctor Alok's program for three years, I am 50 pounds lighter. My taste buds have opened up and I enjoy fresh, wholesome food. Doctor Alok has taught me how to avoid cravings and hunger. It feels good to have control over my eating. I have been able to stay on the program in spite of long hours at work and through the ups and downs of everyday life. If I slip, as I occasionally do, the program allows me get back up, dust myself off and keep on going. This program has been the weight loss answer I had been looking for.

62-year-old female—nursing professional

On Doctor Alok's program, I have lost 25 lbs. over the past two years— and I am still losing weight. This program has given me the tools to work with my body and make healthy eating an enjoyable way of life. If I slip, the program helps me quickly get back on track. I am not hungry, and I have learned to surround myself with better food choices so as to not re-ignite my cravings. I'm not DIEting anymore, I'm finally LIVing. Thank you, Doctor Alok!

43-year-old—mother of five children

I have been on Doctor Alok's program for three years. I lost 30 lbs. in the first year, which is all I needed to lose, and I have kept the weight off ever since. Doctor Alok's program is different from every diet I had tried before. I now understand what causes my hunger and cravings, how my body uses different kinds of food, and how my metabolism affects my weight. I eat healthy and tasty food, and the program allows me to cheat a couple of times a week. What more could one ask for?

55-year-old female—homemaker, church and community volunteer

I have been following Doctor Alok's program for three years. It has been a life-changer for me. I reached my goal weight in four months and have kept the weight off ever since. I am eating healthier, truly enjoying my food, and celebrating my new lower-weight lifestyle! Also, my doctor has cut back on my blood pressure and cholesterol medications.

65-year-old female—interior decorator

Don't take dieting advice from a skinny person

Don't take dieting advice from a skinny person

Doctor Alok's guide to overcoming food addiction and finally losing weight

Alok Kalia MD

ISBN: 1499378718
ISBN 13: 9781499378719
Library of Congress Control Number: 2013922853
CreateSpace Independent Publishing Platform
North Charleston, South Carolina

This book is available at special quantity discounts to use as premiums and sales promotions, or for use in corporate training programs. For more information contact Alok Kalia at
akalia@bluebonnethealth.com

Disclaimer

The author is not your physician and has no professional relationship with you.

The material presented in this book is for education. It is not a substitute for medical counseling.

Before beginning this program, talk to your health care provider about

a) whether this program is right for you,

b) your medical condition,

c) the types of exercise that are suitable for you, and

d) any change in the dosage of medications that might become necessary with the change in eating habits and weight.

Do not stop or change any prescription medication or course of treatment without the approval of your health care provider.

You assume sole responsibility for following any or all of the recommendations in this book.

This book is dedicated to all who have participated in my weight management program over the years. Your shared experience continues to shape this program and make it ever better.

You are my teachers.

Acknowledgements

I want to thank

Robin Stanaland, Kris Kwalik, and Sharon Duncan—
three friends and mentors who said, "You need to write a
book" and then made me do it.

Jerry Boyle, another friend and mentor, who held me
gently accountable and kept me moving forward.

Susan Rapley, RD, for being a collaborator and sounding
board in the critical early years of the program.

Liz Goodgold for making me a more effective writer.
Thank you, Liz.

Henry Devries for his guidance and encouragement.

Sharron Stockhausen for her superb editing.

Everyone who reviewed the manuscript—your critiques
and suggestions were invaluable.

Most of all, I want to thank Raj Kalia, MD—my wife of
four decades, my best friend, my muse.

Table of Contents

Introduction

More than two-thirds of adults in the United States are over-weight—that's 150 million people. Are you one of them?

If so, then you know the answer to weight loss is to eat right and exercise. You try to do just that, over and over again.

But you can't lose the pounds. You blame yourself—"I'm not trying hard enough; I don't do enough exercise; I don't have enough self-control."

The eat-right-and-exercise approach sounds so logical. If eating too many calories makes you gain too many pounds, then taking care of the calories should take care of the pounds. But it does not, either for you or almost anyone else. Here's a thought—if the eat-right-and-exercise answer is not working for 150 million people, *could it be the answer is wrong?*

It is.

The eat-right-and-exercise mantra does not work for so many of us because it ignores the real problem. We don't need to be told to manage our calories—we know that already. But we are not able to do this except for short periods, because food talks to us. Food has power over us. Food tempts us until our cravings overcome our self-control and the weight comes back. Telling us how to manage our calories is not enough—we need to be told how to manage our *cravings.*

How many times have you started a new diet and watched the weight come off, only to see it come right back—often with a few extra pounds tacked on? You know the weight is coming back because you are no longer sticking to the eating plan, but there is nothing you can do about it. A small slip today, another little slip tomorrow, and soon you have lost control over your food choices—yet again.

If you cannot resist putting certain foods into your body even though you are overwhelmed by guilt and regret as you do so, that's a sign of addiction. The first step towards successful, life-long weight management is to understand and overcome this addiction—the cravings and compulsions that lead to the failure of diet after diet. If only the cravings were gone, sticking to the eating plan would be so much easier.

In this book, as the first step, you will learn to manage your hunger and cravings. There is a reason why the body generates hunger, why it craves certain foods. By understanding your body's instincts, its needs and desires, you will be able to make it a partner in your weight loss efforts instead of having it fight you tooth and nail at every turn.

Once you gain control over your hunger and cravings, you are ready to move forwards. You will start on a sensible healthy eating and weight-loss program that is based on the most up-to-date research. You will set a realistic, achievable, and sustainable weight-loss goal. You will learn new ways of cooking and eating. You will recognize and overcome the challenges and temptations that are an unavoidable part of the weight-loss journey. As the weeks and months go by, you will live your new life with increasing confidence and grace.

As the final step in your weight-loss journey, you will set an even more ambitious goal—taking charge of your health. You will partner with your physician to accept responsibility for your blood pressure, blood sugar, and cholesterol levels. Your new understanding of the connections between your eating habits, weight, and health will become the guiding principle in your life.

This book is based on my forty years of experience as a physician, medical school professor, and scientist. I am also one of you; I had to become a specialist in weight loss for the sake of my own health. I understand the challenges you face.

Your journey will take you down a healthier path for the rest of your life. As you look back ten, twenty, thirty years from now, I hope you will be able to say, "Thank you, Dr. Alok!"

Alok Kalia, MD

Part 1:

Getting Ready To Win The Weight-Loss Challenge

Chapter 1

Food Addiction—
"Why Can't I Stop My Hand?"

As a formerly obese physician, let me describe a scene I lived through over and over again.

I am standing in front of a refrigerator. Inside that refrigerator is an apple pie with a flaky crust and oh-so-delicious filling. The pie is sending out waves of attraction that have lured me off the sofa and into the kitchen, staring at the closed door that stands between me and that pie.

I'm not hungry; I've just had dinner. But I know that I am going to eat a piece of that pie. I feel guilty about it, and I should. I am a physician and I am overweight. I, more than most people, know I will harm myself by eating that pie. But I have no choice. My craving for the pie has pushed aside all rational thought. My hand reaches for the refrigerator door.

Why can't I stop my hand?

Have you been an actor in a similar scene? Did you also eat the pie, or the cake, or donut, or pizza? Of course you did.

Why couldn't you stop your hand?

The hand is the problem, is it not? Weight-loss experts and dietitians give us lists of foods to eat and foods to avoid. But no

1

list can help us lose weight. What we really need to know is this: *How do I stop my hand?* No diet will work until we can stop eating the wrong foods in spite of knowing better.

Repeating a potentially harmful behavior against one's better judgment is one of the features of addiction. As you shall see in the next few pages, being addicted to food is not quite the same as being addicted to a drug, but it is close. That is why the simplistic eat-this-not-that approach of most diets does not work. Those diets assume people can choose what to eat and what to avoid. But food addiction, like every other addiction, induces cravings that overcome the ability to make the right choices.

To understand food addiction, we need to ask a basic question: *Why do we eat?* What induces us to put food in our mouths? Let's take a quick look at the answer for now; we will explore it more detail in chapters 3, 4, and 5.

We eat for two reasons—hunger and desire. Of course, we also eat when depressed or stressed or celebrating or partying with friends. But these are occasional reasons for eating. Hunger and desire are the two reasons for eating that are always with us. Both of these are normal, and each serves a different purpose.

The goal of eating for hunger is to replace the calories and nutrients that have been used up in day-to-day living. But eating just enough food to satisfy hunger is not a good survival strategy—it will not help us build a reserve of calories in case food becomes hard to find.

This is exactly the danger our distant ancestors faced. They had no farms or cattle. They lived at the mercy of nature, which meant their food supply was not assured. Even after humans took up farming, crop failure from drought or infestation was a constant threat. To survive periods of food scarcity, they had to eat extra calories whenever these were available, hungry or not, so their bodies could make and store some fat. This may be why we are programmed to find calorie-rich food so desirable that we will eat it even when not hungry. "Never walk by easy calories without eating some" is the motto of the body, and this approach served us well for most of our existence.

But something has changed. Until recently, every high-calorie food was a *natural* food. Natural foods are attractive, but they do not induce cravings that compel us into acting irrationally. Even if I desire a natural food, it is not an overwhelming desire. I like apples, but I can say no to an apple without thinking twice about it. When dealing with natural high-calorie foods, I am able to maintain a balance between *attraction* and *restraint*.

But today we have the ability create "designer" foods that are ever more appealing to the taste buds. Designer foods are foods that are immensely tastier than the components from which they are made. For most of human existence, we ate the components. But think of ice cream or chocolate cake or pizza or chips; think of your favorite menu items in your favorite restaurant; look at the recipes in any cookbook. These foods are so tasty because they are fine-tuned to our palates to a degree nature cannot achieve—these foods are *unnaturally* tasty. In fact, the way we turn natural foods into designer foods is similar to how we turn coca leaves into crack cocaine.

Cocaine is naturally present in the leaves of the coca plant. The native people of South America have chewed coca leaves for thousands of years. Chewing the leaves is mildly stimulating but not addictive because there is only a very small amount of cocaine in each leaf. But when we extract and concentrate the cocaine from a pile of coca leaves into a crystal of crack cocaine, it becomes highly addictive. We have done the same thing with our food—we have learned to extract and concentrate tastes, and by doing so made food highly addictive.

We are now surrounded by this unnatural but very tasty food that upsets the balance between attraction and restraint. Eating such food creates a wave of pleasure. The pleasurable experience of yesterday is not quite forgotten before the same pleasure is experienced again today. These repeated waves of pleasure begin to elevate normal desire into abnormal cravings that make us behave irrationally. Have you ever made an ice cream run at 10 p.m.? Eaten a donut while consumed by guilt? Downed four slices of pizza even though you intended to have only one?

All of these are signs of addiction—your food is now beginning to control you. Psychiatrists list seven behaviors that point to addiction; a diagnosis of addiction can be made if a person exhibits any *three* of these in the past twelve months. The behaviors are:

1. Taking in more of the substance than was originally intended.
2. Failing over and over again to use less of the substance.
3. Going out of the way to obtain the substance.
4. Continuing to use the substance in spite of knowing it is causing harm.
5. Having withdrawal symptoms.
6. Giving up social, occupational, or recreational activities because of use of the substance.
7. Needing to use more and more of the substance to get the same effect.

Replace the words "the substance" with "my favorite foods." Do three or more of these behaviors apply to you? I would bet many overweight people can identify with numbers one through four on this list. This is the reason terms such as "chocoholic" and "falling off the wagon" have long been part of the weight-loss vocabulary.

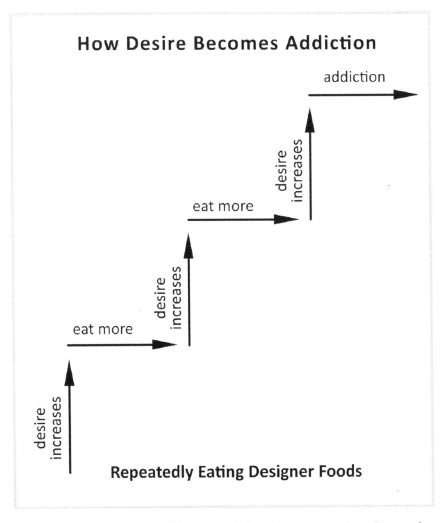

Figure 1. Highly tasty "designer" foods elevate the desire for high-calorie foods (which is normal) into food addiction (which is not).

Addiction takes away the ability to make choices about the addictive substance. Unfortunately, all diets demand choice, so there is tension—what the body craves is different from what the diet allows. In the first few weeks of a diet, the weight comes off quickly and the sheer joy of seeing the needle on the scale move in the desired direction makes it possible to suppress one's cravings. But then the weight loss slows. The needle moves less and less, and on some days it does not move at all. The high of

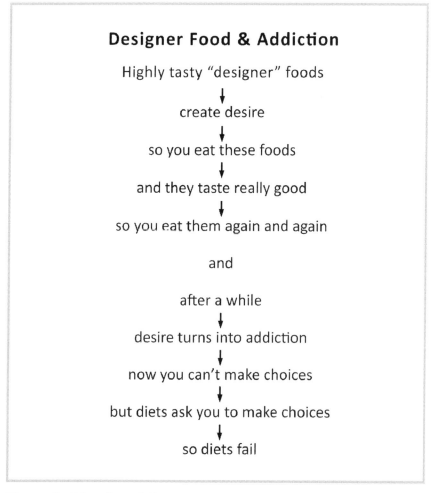

Figure 2. Why diets fail.

the first few weeks gives way to frustration. When that happens, cravings become harder to resist. Non-regulation foods begin to creep back on the menu. A little cheating today, a little more tomorrow, and soon the addiction is back. Another diet bites the dust.

Any eating plan that is sustainable in the long run must start by eliminating the cravings, by overcoming food addiction. Fortunately, this is not difficult. Addiction to food is not like addiction to alcohol or cocaine or heroin or nicotine. These are "hard" addictions, caused by chemicals that have no normal function in the body. These chemicals grab on to the desire mechanisms and won't let go, so de-addiction is difficult.

Food addiction, in contrast, is a soft addiction; it is just an intensification of normal desire caused by today's highly tasty designer foods, an intensification of the inherent instinct to make and store fat. Food addiction is relatively easy to switch off. Just remove unnatural, highly tasty, designer foods from the plate and the addiction disappears within a few days. Most people who faithfully follow the program in this book are de-addicted within a week. Once the cravings are gone, making the right choices becomes so much easier.

Of course, in today's food environment the danger of becoming re-addicted is extremely high. Addiction—any addiction—has been compared to a tiger that has you in its jaws. When you are trying to overcome a drug addiction, you can lock the tiger in the cage, walk away, and fight your cravings until they are gone. But you cannot walk away from food—you have to eat, and every meal offers an opportunity to become re-addicted. You lock the tiger in the cage—but you have to take it out three times a day for a walk. If you are not careful, it will clamp its jaws on you again. This book shows you how to walk the tiger without being bitten.

Comfort Food?

In today's food environment, making good choices requires a clear mind that is brimming with emotional energy. If you are mentally exhausted, there is no energy left to draw upon.

A stressful day at work, a difficult and draining relationship, the loss of a loved one—all these can leave you running on empty. You have no energy left to make the hard choices that are necessary for eating correctly. Out comes the ice cream or pizza or fried chicken. We call these "comfort foods" because they temporarily provide a bit of pleasure to counteract the fatigue and depression. In the long run, though, comfort foods add weight, impact health, and just make us uncomfortable.

Doctor Alok says:

- Our distant ancestors did not have an assured food supply, so they had to eat calorie-rich foods whenever available in order to make and store fat.
- This instinctive desire for high-calorie foods is still with us.
- In the past, all high-calorie foods were natural foods such as sweet fruits and starchy roots. These foods are attractive but not addictive.

- Now we can turn natural foods into highly tasty artificial foods—ice cream, pizza, chocolate cake. These "designer" foods are tastier than anything nature can produce.
- These highly tasty foods elevate desire (which is normal) into food addiction (which is not).
- The cravings induced by food addiction make it extremely difficult to stay on a diet.
- The first step in successful weight management is to eliminate food addiction.
- De-addiction from food is not difficult and can be done fairly quickly.

Chapter 2

Don't Take Dieting Advice from a Skinny Person

A person who has never been heavy cannot fully comprehend the enormous power that food has over the rest of us.

People are different from each other. Not everyone is equally susceptible to becoming addicted to food, just as not everyone is equally susceptible to becoming addicted to a drug. For example, about 12 percent of the population of the United States is susceptible to alcohol addiction. Even though alcohol is freely available, this number is quite stable. To put it another way, if we were to encourage one hundred people who had never tasted alcohol to have a few drinks every day, twelve are at risk of becoming addicted to alcohol while the other eighty-eight are not. Of course, this number applies only to the population as a whole; the susceptibility appears to be different in people of different ethnic backgrounds.

Food addiction appears to work in the same way; it seems that about two-thirds of us are at risk. The percentage of overweight adults in the USA increased rapidly between 1975 and 2000, from about 40 percent to 66 percent and then leveled off. In the following ten years it increased hardly at all, from 66 percent to 69 percent. During that decade there was not a great change either in the societal attitudes towards obesity or in types of food that were available. So if we use the alcohol model, this leveling off would suggest that as many as two-thirds of us are susceptible to some degree of food addiction and the other third are not. Also, these numbers are for the population of the United States as a whole; in certain ethnic groups the percentage of overweight people is much higher.

The lower susceptibility to food addiction might be one reason why a third of all adults are able to stay at a normal weight without too much effort; food just does not call out to them as it does to the rest of us.

There is always tension between the call of the addictive substance and the degree of restraint a person can exert. People who are less susceptible to the call of food need less restraint. In these individuals, the rational mind is almost always in control so they can make better food choices and maintain a normal body weight. These people are not thin because they have more self-control; *they are thin because they require less self-control,* because their desires do not turn into addictive cravings. For them, eating correctly is easier than it is for the rest of us. Of course, some people also seem to have a faster metabolism—they store fewer calories as fat, so they can eat all they want and not gain a pound.

So when we see all those skinny people in TV infomercials telling us how to lose weight, remember—they live in one world, we live in another. They cannot show us how to stop our hands, because their hands rarely betray them.

I believe the most important questions to ask a weight-loss expert are: Have you personally lost weight? Were you obese before you became thin? If the answer is no, then the person may not understand the role that food addiction plays in your life and mine. I suspect that many weight-loss experts are not attracted to food like the rest of us, which may be why most weight-loss programs focus only on "eat this, not that" while ignoring the critical challenge of food addiction. Unfortunately, this is also why most weight-loss programs ultimately fail.

Doctor Alok says:

- People seem to have differing susceptibility to food addiction.
- Those who are not susceptible to food addiction find it easier to stay thin.
- A person who has never been heavy cannot fully understand the power that food has over those who are, or have been, heavy.

Chapter 3

The Reasons for Eating:
Hunger and Desire

In chapter 1 you read about the effect of food addiction on eating behavior. However, food addiction is an unnatural urge created by unnatural foods. To be able to gain control over eating, you also need to understand the natural urges for eating. What are these natural urges?

There are two: hunger and desire, and they have entirely different goals. The goal of *hunger* is to replace the calories that have been used up in the course of staying alive and carrying out everyday activities such as walking, talking, and working; the goal of *desire* is to encourage us to take in extra calories and store them as fat for future use.

These two different reasons to eat served us well when we were dependent on nature for our food. In the northern hemisphere, for example, in spring and early summer there was probably just enough food (lots of leaves but no ripe fruits); in late summer and early fall food was plentiful (ripe fruits, roots, and wild game); and winter was a period of scarcity, a time to hunker down and survive. Each of these situations calls for a different food-gathering and eating strategy.

When there is just enough food, it makes sense to use hunger as the main stimulus for eating, to focus on replacing the calories that have been used. I call this the "replacement" mode. The goal is to eat enough so as to not lose weight, but make no effort to store fat. Making fat requires eating an excess of calories. If there is just enough food available, walking around trying to find excess food is likely to use up more calories with no guarantee of success. It's simply not a good survival strategy.

But when food is plentiful and excess calories such as tasty fruits are readily available, it makes sense to switch into the fat-making mode. To make fat, we need to eat more than just replacement calories; we need to eat beyond hunger. Now desire (instead of hunger) becomes the stimulus for eating. Desire will make you eat whether you are hungry or not. When you start eating lunch at a restaurant, your goal is to satisfy your hunger. But by the time the waiter brings out the dessert tray, you are no longer hungry. If you decide to have the cheesecake, you are clearly responding to desire, not hunger.

As you saw in chapter 1, we are programmed to find high-calorie foods attractive, to desire such foods. When the body sees lots of such foods available, it goes into the fat-making mode. When you are in this mode, you will constantly think about and seek desirable foods. You will eat for hunger, and then you will overeat for desire.

There are also times when food is scarce. That's when you tap into the fat stores that were laid up during the good times. Something else also happens; when fat is being used as the main source of energy, chemicals called "ketones" flood the system. Ketones suppress hunger. This makes sense; if the body is drawing on its fat stores, there *must* be a shortage of food—and if there is a shortage of food, there is no point in making you hungry. In the next two chapters, I will explore hunger and desire in more detail.

Doctor Alok says:

- The goal of *hunger* is to replace the calories that have been used.
- The goal of *desire* is to eat extra calories and make fat.

Chapter 4

Eating for Hunger:
My Stomach is Growling!

When the food supply is adequate but not excessive, humans maintain a remarkably steady body weight. This means there is a balance between calories used and calories eaten. How do you know how much to eat? After all, you do not weigh yourself before sitting down at the table and then eat just the right number of calories.

Actually, that *is* what you do; you just don't know you are doing it. Your body keeps track of your weight and knows how many calories you need to keep from losing weight. It does not try to balance out the calories at every meal—after all, hunter-gatherers had no control over how much food was available at each meal. But, over the course of days and weeks, the body does a remarkable job of balancing calories used and calories eaten. It does this by sensing the need for calories, then generating hunger until that need is satisfied—but not beyond.

For our distant ancestors, hunting and gathering was just the start. Food had to be cleaned, cut, shelled, husked, pounded, and cooked over an open fire. The work and the danger involved in finding and preparing food acted as a counterbalance to hunger. A person had to be hungry enough to do the work needed to find enough food, but as soon as hunger was satisfied the need for finding food disappeared.

Hunger is regulated by complex internal mechanisms. When the stomach is empty, it makes a hormone called *ghrelin*. Ghrelin gets into the blood, goes to a "hunger center" in the brain, and lets it know the stomach is empty. The hunger center knows it's time to generate hunger—but how much?

What is a Hormone?

A hormone is a chemical that is produced in one part of the body, then taken by the blood to distant places to do its thing. Testosterone is made in the testes, but it makes the beard grow. Thyroid hormone is made by a gland in the neck, but it regulates the metabolism of every cell in the body. Insulin is produced by the pancreas (an organ that sits behind the stomach), but regulates the entry of glucose in cells all the way from the scalp to the big toe. Similarly, ghrelin is produced by the stomach and has its effect in the brain.

The hunger center receives messages from the stomach, but it also keeps track of the body weight by keeping an eye on the fat stores. Aside from childhood and old age (and in bodybuilders), any change in body weight is usually caused by an increase or decrease in body fat. So what the hunger center really does is keep track of the amount of fat in the body. The job of the hunger center is to keep the body fat (and therefore the body weight) constant.

Fat makes a hormone called *leptin*. The level of leptin in the blood depends on the amount of fat in the body. As the amount of body fat increases, so does the leptin level. As the amount of fat decreases, the leptin level goes down. The hunger center keeps track of body weight by following the trend in the leptin level. If the level is going down, the person must be using up the stored fat, which means the number of calories coming is not enough to replace those being used up – and this means the person is not eating enough. Perhaps food is getting hard to find? The hunger center increases the hunger level to try and make the person work harder at finding food.

The cruise control and the rubber band

Between the ghrelin, leptin, and the hunger center, the body weight can be kept amazingly stable from month to month and year to year. This ability of the body to keep things the same is known as *homeostasis*. The body has many homeostatic mechanisms, and each has a set point. For example, body temperature is maintained by a homeostatic mechanism with a set point of 98.6 degrees F. Go outside in the cold without warm clothes, and you will soon start to shiver. Your muscles have been ordered to generate heat to prevent your body temperature from falling. Go jogging in the hot sun, and the homeostatic mechanism will make you sweat;

evaporation of the sweat cools you off and prevents you from overheating.

The Cruise Control

The cruise control in your car functions like a homeostatic mechanism. The speed you set is the set point. The cruise control increases or decreases the flow of fuel to the engine and manipulates the engine controls to keep the speed at that set point.

Body weight also seems to have a set point. Unlike the set point for temperature, however, the set point for body weight seems to work only in one direction. It will try and stop you from losing weight, but will happily step aside and let you gain weight. This made perfect sense when humans lived in the jungle—the more fat a person could put on when food was plentiful, the greater the chance of surviving if food became hard to find. Of course, the opportunities to make fat were few and far between, so obesity was never an issue. The body only needed a one-way set point, so that's what it has.

Weight-loss studies consistently show that when a person who has lost weight falls off the wagon, the tendency is to go back towards the weight at the start of the weight loss. This suggests the set point for body weight is the person's highest recent weight. Also, when a person gains weight and stays at the new, higher, weight for a while, the new weight becomes the new set point. Recent medical studies that have tracked ghrelin and leptin levels after weight loss seem to support this theory.

What a bummer! Well, perhaps not. Can the set point move down under the right conditions? What happens to the set point if a person loses weight and then stays at the lower weight for some months or a year or more? There is not yet enough research on this to give a clear answer, but the experience in our clinic's weight-loss program seems to suggest that after a while the set point begins to come down. If a person can stay at the lower weight for a while, then even if that person starts regaining weight, he or she will not quickly go back to the original weight because the set point is now lower. Although it's not known how long it takes to lower the set point, it is clearly more than just a few months.

To put it another way, imagine you are holding one end of a rubber band tightly between the thumb and forefinger of your left hand and the other end a little more loosely between the thumb and forefinger of your right hand. The left hand is

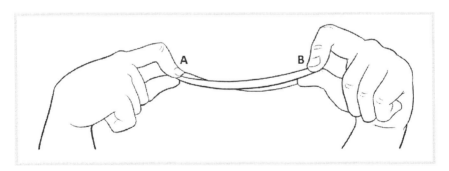

Figure 3. When the set point for weight (A) and the current weight (B) are the same, there is no tension in the rubber band.

your body-weight set point and the right hand is your current weight. If your current weight is the same as your set point, there is no tension in the rubber band.

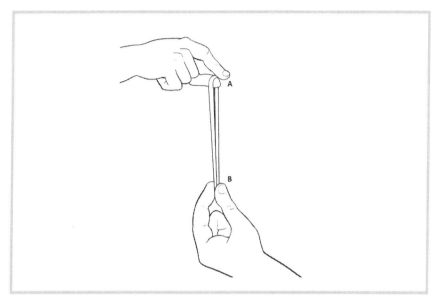

Figure 4. As you start losing weight, the rubber band is stretched more and more.

But as you begin to lose weight, your right hand goes down and the rubber band starts to stretch. Now there is tension. If you lose too much weight too quickly, the rubber band is stretched too tight; it is likely to slip from your right hand and snap back.

But if you gently lose a moderate amount of weight, you will create only a gentle stretch and you will be able to hold on to the rubber band with your right hand. As the months go by, the stretch in the rubber band will gradually pull your left hand downwards. *You have reset the set point.* That is your goal.

The Rebound from Weight Loss

When you rebound from weight loss, you often end up weighing more than when you started. One reason is that rapid weight loss causes muscle loss. This is bad, because the muscles are one of the biggest users of calories. The other reason is that rapid weight loss forces the body to slow down its metabolism so the body can make do with fewer calories.

If you fall off the wagon and go back to eating the same number of calories as before, guess what? The body learned to use fewer calories so even more of them will be stored as fat.

Doctor Alok says:

- When food is adequate but not plentiful, the hunger center in the brain keeps the body weight remarkably constant.
- The hunger center receives signals both from the stomach ("I am empty") and from the body's storage depots (either "all is well" or "fat is disappearing").
- Depending on the fat storage situation, the hunger center decides how much hunger to generate—a little bit or a lot.
- The body fights weight loss, but is always happy to see weight gain because fat is insurance against famine.

Chapter 5

Eating for Desire:
My Mouth is Watering!

Eating to satisfy hunger and maintain a stable body weight is fine if there is always enough food available. But what happens if there is a shortage of food that goes on for weeks or months? The best way to survive such scarcity is to have a good supply of fat on board. Eating only to satisfy hunger may prevent weight loss, but it will not help us make and store the fat we may need for survival. For this we have to eat for a different reason: desire.

As the old one-liner goes, "I am not fat; I am just better prepared for the coming famine!"

We are naturally programmed to desire high-calorie foods, to find them attractive. What would you rather eat: a piece of broccoli or a slice of ripe, sweet, juicy, honeydew melon? The melon, of course. I would too, and so would almost everyone else. Finding a melon more attractive than broccoli is hard-wired into our system. We are attracted to foods that contain excess calories because they can easily be converted into fat.

Along with the hunger center, you also have an "appetite center" that responds to pleasure *and to the prospect of pleasure.*

This prospect of pleasure creates *desire;* it creates a connection between the food and you. The desire to eat attractive foods has nothing to do with hunger. Hunger will make you eat, but desire will make you overeat. It is desire that makes you order dessert even after your stomach is full. Hunger pushes you towards food. "Go eat something, anything!" says hunger. Desirable food pulls you towards itself. "Come eat me!" says the desirable food.

Hunger *vs.* Desire

Hunger and desire really are different. Hunger makes your stomach growl; desire makes your mouth water. *Desire never makes your stomach growl; hunger never makes your mouth water.* Think about this the next time you are getting ready to eat something. What is driving you to the food? Is it your stomach, or is it your mouth?

Before humanity started farming and keeping livestock, calorie-rich, fat-producing foods were available only at some times during the year. As you read in the previous chapter, for those living in the northern hemisphere, summer and early fall were the best eating times—fruits were ripe and game was abundant. To survive the oncoming winter, it was crucial to gorge on these foods and make as much fat as possible. So people would put on fat in the summer and fall (eating for desire), use the fat to survive the winter, and try to hold their own in the spring (eating for hunger). Then the cycle started again. Other parts of the world experience different year-round eating cycles, but periods of plenty often alternate with periods when less food is available.

If the goal is to make fat, which foods provide the most calories per bite? Those should be the foods we most desire. There are two types of nutrients that can easily be turned into fat. The first, of course, is fat itself. The second is carbohydrate, or carbs—sugar and starch. By the way, excess protein calories are not turned into fat.

Carbohydrates seem to be our primary desirable food. We love sugar and starch. Ripe fruits and starchy roots (think potatoes) are attractive. Melon and pineapple and luscious pears; berries and oranges and sweet grapes—yum!

What about fat? Fat is a richer source of calories than carbs. An ounce of fat has twice as many calories as an ounce of carbohydrate. Interestingly, humans (unlike laboratory rats) don't seem to crave fat by itself. How often do you slink into the kitchen at night and drink a bottle of oil? Do you lick unsalted butter or snack on a chunk of lard? Most people don't.

In fact, humans don't even have taste buds for fat. Sweet, sour, salt, bitter, yes, and even umami, the newly discovered taste sensation for savory foods. But there are no obvious taste buds for fat. Instead, we detect fat by its texture. We say that something is oily or buttery. Oily is a texture, not a taste. You don't have to put a drop of oil in your mouth to know it is oily— you can get the same information by rubbing a drop between finger and thumb. But you cannot detect saltiness or sweetness with your finger and thumb.

Why don't we desire fat in the same way we desire carbs? One reason might be that compared to carbs, fat is not plentiful in the jungle. Wild animals tend to be lean, and most plant products are not detectably fatty. Nuts have oil, but it is not easy to extract the oil without machinery. And, of course, hunter-gatherers had no butter because they had no cattle. So fruits and roots might have been a better calorie-rich prize to focus on than fat.

Of course, in today's world, we can produce all the butter and oil we want, and now we do desire fat, but for a different reason. We desire fat because it is a wonderful carrier of flavor. Fat extracts flavor from food and delivers it to the taste buds. Fat intensifies the taste of other foods. Fat can even make flavors float in the air—the smell of sizzling bacon fills the whole house. Fat also make the texture of food so much more appealing. The moistness of a cake, the flakiness of a croissant – it is the magic of fat that makes those things happen. Fat makes it so easy to turn ordinary food into designer food. We love to add fat to our food to enhance its flavor, its texture, its "mouth feel," and we love to fry things in fat.

So we *do* love fat, but only as a companion to other foods, not for itself. From the obesity perspective, if we can stay away from carbs, we will automatically stay away from fat *because we do not eat fat without carbs*. Think of carbs as the bank robber; fat just drives the getaway car. Fat facilitates the crime. But if there is no robber in the bank, the getaway car can do no harm. Beware of the carbs!

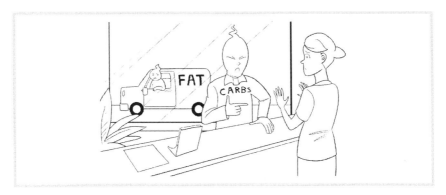

Figure 5. Carbs are the bank robbers; fat drives the getaway car.

Doctor Alok says:

- To survive when food is in short supply, we need to make and store fat ahead of time.
- We are programmed to desire and eat high-calorie foods whenever available, even if the stomach is full. This is the only sure way to make fat.
- The foods we seem to most desire are carbs—sugar and starch. We also desire fat but only because it make other foods taste better. We do not eat fat by itself.

Part 2:

What's Your Weight-Loss Goal?

Chapter 6

A Sensible Approach to Weight Loss

There are two common reasons for trying to lose weight. The first is to improve your health; the second is to improve your appearance. The two, of course, go hand in hand, but it is important to decide up front which is the more important. This decision will affect both your weight-loss journey and your sense of whether you have succeeded or failed.

So—why do *you* want to lose weight? If your answer is "I want to look better," then you will judge your success by the change in your appearance. If this is your goal, there is no limit to the amount of weight you will want to lose. You might start by saying, "I want to lose just ten pounds." However, when you reach that goal, the temptation is to lose a little more, and then a little more, and to lose it as quickly as possible because you love the way your face and your body are changing.

But there is a risk in going down this road. If you lose too much weight too quickly, your body will fight back. You may find yourself falling off the wagon and regaining the weight. In fact, you may end up heavier than you were when you started because of muscle loss and slower metabolism that can result from losing weight too quickly (see The Rebound from Weight Loss in chapter 4).

On the other hand, if your answer is, "I want to make a measurable and long-lasting improvement in my health," then your approach will be different. You will set a weight-loss goal based on sound medical principles, and you will reach and maintain the goal. Your focus will be on keeping off the weight you lost.

You will also not go on a diet. Many popular diets force you into imbalanced eating with too much of some foods and not enough of others. Some diets also reduce the food intake to a starvation level. For most people, these unnatural eating patterns might be great for losing weight quickly but cannot be sustained for months and years.

If you are trying to lose weight for life-long health improvement, you need to take the long view and stay away from programs that promise quick results. You need to make simple and sensible changes in the way you shop, cook, and eat. Your goal is to learn to walk with confidence through today's confusing food environment, picking out only what is good for you and ignoring everything else.

The program in this book will help you lose weight and make life-long changes to improve your health. Of course you will also end up looking better, but that is just a side benefit.

To set a rational weight-loss goal, you need to answer three questions:

1. Am I overweight?
2. If so, how much of the excess weight do I need to lose to improve my health?
3. Finally, over what period of time should I lose this weight?

The most common yardstick for defining overweight is the body mass index, or BMI. To calculate the BMI, the height and weight are plugged into a formula (see chapter 7). A person with a BMI of less than 18.5 is considered underweight; 18.5 to 24.9 is normal weight, and 25 to 29.9 is overweight. A BMI of 30 or more is labeled as obesity.

The relationship of BMI to health and disease is not perfect, but studies have shown that, in general, a BMI of more than thirty is a health risk and a reason to lose weight. For those with a BMI less than thirty, the presence of excess belly fat (see next section) or conditions such as high blood pressure, pre-diabetes or type 2 diabetes, heart disease, sleep apnea, etc. also makes weight loss an important part of health improvement.

One criticism of the BMI is that it looks at the weight, but not at what is contributing to the weight. Muscle is heavy, so it is possible for a heavily-muscled bodybuilder to have almost no body fat and still have a high BMI. While this is true, it is probably fair to say that most people reading this book are not Arnold Schwarzenegger look-alikes. For most, a high BMI means the person is carrying too much fat. This is why the BMI is commonly used to define obesity and set weight-loss goals.

Of Apples and Pears

There is another, more important failing of the BMI—while BMI strongly suggests a person is carrying excess fat, it cannot say where in the body the fat is stored. This is important because not all of us store fat in the same places, and all fat is not equally harmful to health.

On the road to weight gain, most people start by collecting fat in and around the abdomen. This excess fat around the middle results in an "apple" shape. Others collect excess fat in the hips and thighs; this is called the "pear" shape. The difference is important. As far as diabetes, heart disease, fatty liver, and even sleep apnea are concerned, only the fat in and around the belly seems to matter. In contrast, fat in the hips and thighs seems to have few, if any medical consequences. So, the apple shape is considered to be a lot more harmful than the pear shape. Of course, a person may start out pear-shaped and then collect fat around the middle or "add an apple above the pear." If this occurs, the person incurs the same medical risk as any as any other apple-shaped person.

What is so special about belly fat? The abdomen is nature's preferred place to store fat, as is so often brought to our notice when the pants become tight around the waist. Belly fat is active fat—it stays in constant communication with the rest of the body, always ready and willing to dissolve itself and serve as a source of calories if food is in short supply. For this reason, when a person starts to lose weight, the belly fat often melts away more quickly than fat in other parts of the body.

Belly fat played an important role in helping our ancestors survive famine, increasing in amount when the food was plentiful and getting used up when food became scarce. Fortunately—or unfortunately—for most of us food is always plentiful and the balance between making fat and using fat has been lost. There is rarely a reason to tap into the store. As a result, we collect fat an excessive amount of fat around the middle.

Think of a messy, overstuffed closet, disorganized and bursting at the seams. One day you open the doors, look at the mess, and say, "I can't take it anymore!" You just wade in there and start throwing stuff out. Something similar seems to happen in the abdomen. If the amount of fat in the belly becomes excessive, the body starts to do a little housecleaning. Some of the fat cells begin to degenerate and white blood cells come in to clean up the mess.

Whenever white cells become activated, whether they are fighting bacteria or removing dead tissue, the result is inflammation. With the entry of these active white cells, scattered areas of inflammation develop throughout the belly fat. This is a very low-grade inflammation with no pain, no fever, and no redness. But what this inflammation lacks in intensity, it makes up in persistence. It goes on month after month, year after year.

Inflammation serves a purpose. Inflammation is how the body fights infection. When you have a sore throat, your body is using inflammation to fight the invading bacteria and white blood cells are its frontline troops. As the cells swing into action, they release chemicals into the blood that tell the rest of the body to get on a war footing. Your temperature rises, your heart speeds up, your immune system goes into high gear. You are alert, ready, and poised for a fight. This is good because it helps you overcome the infection. But continuous and misdirected inflammation can be harmful. The body can stay on a war footing only so long before its normal activities are disturbed. This is what seems to result from the prolonged, low-grade inflammation going on in the belly fat. Even though the amount of chemicals seeping out is small, over the course of months and years these chemicals begin to have harmful health effects.

Is there a yardstick to directly measure the belly fat? There is, and it is called the waist circumference—literally, how big you are around the waist. There are numbers for normal and abnormal waist circumference in men and women of different ethnicities, but it is not really necessary to know these numbers. If you are bigger around your waist than you are around your hips, you likely have too much belly fat. Another simple trick is to stand up straight and look down the middle, bending only your neck. If you can't see your toes because your abdomen is in the way, you need to think about losing weight, regardless of your BMI.

Belly fat is bad, but there is some good news too. As you read just a few paragraphs ago, "When a person starts to lose weight, the belly fat melts away more quickly than fat in other parts of the body." Even a small decrease in the belly fat begins to turn off the inflammation. For this reason, a weight loss of just 10 percent yields a great health benefit. In fact, many obesity researchers consider a 5 percent weight loss a success, but 10 percent is a safer bet.

Doctor Alok says:

- A BMI of more than thirty increases the risk of health problems.
- Excess belly fat, regardless of the BMI, increases the risk of health problems.
- A small, sustained weight loss is enough to provide long-lasting health benefits.

Chapter 7

Setting Your Personal Weight-Loss Goal

Now you are ready to set your weight-loss goal, using your BMI as the yardstick. You can find your BMI by going to *http://www.nhlbi. nih.gov/guidelines/obesity/BMI/bmicalc.htm* or any of the other BMI calculators available on the Internet; all you need to do is to put in your height and weight. If you don't have Internet access or are mathematically inclined, the BMI is the (weight in lbs. X 703) / (height in inches)^2 OR the (weight in kg.) / (height in meters)^2.

If your BMI is higher than thirty-five, your weight loss goal should be 10-15 percent of your starting weight. The first 10 percent of the weight loss will help your blood sugar level, your blood pressure, and your heart. However, at this level of BMI, there is also a lot of wear and tear on your hips, knees, and ankles from the excess weight and losing the extra few percent, if possible, will help to relieve this.

Example:
Height 5' 5"
Current weight 240 lbs.

BMI: 39.9

Since the calculated BMI is more than 35, the weight loss goal will be 10-15 percent of 240, or between 24 and 36 lbs.

If your BMI is between 30 and 35, your weight loss goal will be 10 percent of your starting weight.

Example:
Height 5' 5"
Weight 200 lbs.
BMI: 33.3

Since the calculated BMI is between 30 and 35, the weight loss goal will be 10 percent of 200, or 20 lbs.

If your BMI is between 25 and 29.9, you are still likely to benefit from losing some weight, especially if you carry excess fat around the middle or have medical problems that might improve from weight loss. In this weight range, it is not possible to set a hard target for the weight loss. A good rule of thumb is to first go for a 5 percent weight loss. When this is achieved, decide whether going for another 5 percent is necessary and achievable.

Example:
Height 5' 5"
Weight 170 lbs.
BMI: 28.3

Since the calculated BMI is between 25 and 29.9, the initial weight loss goal would be 5 percent of 170, or 8.5 lbs. If this is achieved relatively easily and without excessive hunger, trying to lose another 8.5 lbs. (for a total weight loss of 17 lbs.) is not unreasonable.

Don't Stretch The Rubber Band!

How fast should you try to lose the weight? The simple answer is: in no less than three months. In fact, if your starting BMI is more than thirty-five, then taking four to six months to reach your goal is not unreasonable.

Why at least three months? In chapter 4 I talked about the rubber band that is attached at one end to your starting weight and at the other end to your new, lower weight. As your weight goes down, the rubber band stretches. Stretch it too quickly, and it will slip through your fingers and snap back.

The body loses weight reluctantly because it is being asked to give up its fat, its savings. You have to take your body by the hand and gently lead it down the road to weight loss. You have to sweet-talk it, cajole it into coming along. Start pulling too hard and the body will stubbornly dig in its heels and fight you by making you hungry and slowing your metabolism. This is why a minimum period of three months is a reasonable goal for your weight loss.

Of course, people are different, and it is possible to hit the 10 percent goal much earlier than three months. If this happens to you, there is no need to panic. If you are eating all the meals you should be eating, if you are not skimping on the amount of food at each meal, if you are not thinking constantly about food or having hunger pangs, then just keep going. But if you find you have drifted from eating sensibly into eating less and less in order to lose weight even faster—well, you are yanking on your body and risking a fight. You need to re-evaluate your eating habits. Stop being in such a hurry.

Even if you are not consciously trying to cut back on your eating to lose weight faster, there is a trap you can easily fall into while doing this program. One of the changes many people notice within a few days of starting the program is an almost complete lack of hunger. If this happens, it is easy to forget to eat. Don't do it—it will come back to haunt you. I will talk a lot more about this later on in the book.

Doctor Alok says:

- You should set an achievable and sustainable goal for your weight loss.
- Moderate weight loss leads to long-lasting health benefits.
- Too rapid weight loss increases the risk of regaining the lost weight.

Part 3:

Setting The Stage—
Dr. Alok's
Weight-Loss
Secrets

Everyone knows that the first step in weight management is to eat the right foods while avoiding the wrong foods. For most of us, though, there seems to be an unbridgeable gap between knowing what to do and actually doing it. Eliminating food addiction is a big first step towards bridging this gap, but there is a set of actions, behaviors, and knowledge that will help your odds of losing weight and keeping it off for the rest of your life.

This section is titled "Dr. Alok's Weight-Loss Secrets," but these secrets are based either on well-accepted scientific principles or on plain old common sense. The goal is to make you an expert on your own body. Much of the science may be new to you, but as you read through this section, you will begin to understand how carbs are turned into fat, how you can use the hunger hormone to your advantage, and much more.

The eating program in the next part of the book will show you how to apply this information in real life. For now, just focus on understanding and learning it. Knowing *why* you are doing something makes it more likely that you will do it correctly. So even if you are anxious to start on your weight loss journey, take the time to read through this section. You will never think about food and eating in the same way ever again.

Chapter 8

Secret #1:
Plan Ahead

You should always be one day ahead in your eating. This means you should know today what you will eat tomorrow.

Planning ahead is critical because every meal offers an opportunity to stray. Waiting until you are hungry to make your eating choices is a recipe for disaster.

Making the right choices requires willpower and energy. Each of us starts the day with only so much decision-making energy. Every difficult decision uses up some of this energy, so a hard day at work can leave you drained and exhausted. Add to this the usual ups and downs of life—a rocky personal relationship, a tight financial situation, illness in the family, the loss of a loved one, a teenager who is driving you up the wall—and your store of energy may be exhausted long before the day is done.

When that happens you are in the danger zone. You are hungry, and you no longer have the energy and mental toughness to make the hard eating choices. You push aside your rational mind and reach out for comfort food. Of course, comfort food ultimately leads only to discomfort; it leaves you riddled both with guilt and with fat.

But there is a different approach. What if you didn't have to make any choices? What if you already had a plan in place for each of today's meals, *a plan that you made and committed to memory the previous evening?* When you do that there are no decisions to be made. All you have to do is to follow the plan.

So, every evening, you need to spend a few minutes making an eating plan for the next day. Ask yourself—what will I have for breakfast, lunch, and dinner? What snacks will I eat between meals? Will I be eating out? If so, what type of food will I order and more important, what type of food will I absolutely, positively stay away from?

These decisions need to be made a day ahead and etched in your mind. Writing down your plan is even better. The more concrete your decisions, the greater the odds that you will stick with them, eat correctly, and lose weight.

Because you planned ahead, you will have the food on hand to prepare a quick and healthy breakfast. Your snacks will be packed and ready to go. You already know what you are going to have for lunch. Perhaps most important, you will have made sure there is something healthy and tasty in your refrigerator when you get home the next evening. You know from experience that this is when you are most likely to be exhausted and prone to eating the wrong things.

So—plan ahead. Staying one day ahead in your eating choices will make it much more likely that you will eat what you should be eating. You will begin to win your food-choice battles, and each victory will increase your commitment to eating right and staying healthy. Of all the strategies for healthful eating and weight loss, planning ahead is by far the most important. If you remember only two words after you finish reading this book, I hope those words are *plan ahead*.

Doctor Alok says:

- Every evening, make an eating plan for the next day.
- If you plan today what you are going to eat tomorrow, you are less likely to stray from your eating program even if you are stressed, exhausted, or just plain tempted.

Chapter 9

Secret #2: You Can Control Where Those Calories Go

It seems logical to assume that eating too much fat will make you fat. But eating too much carbohydrate will also make you fat. Of the two, carbohydrates, or carbs are by far the bigger culprit.

Carbs seem to have played a major role in kicking off the obesity epidemic. The 1980s and 1990s saw dramatic increases in the percentage of Americans who were overweight or obese. During this time the percentage of carb calories in the American diet went up and up, while the percentage of fat calories remained fairly steady.

One reason for the increase in carb consumption was the highly-publicized research studies in the early 1970s that pointed to a link between saturated fat and heart disease. Not surprisingly, this lead to a boom in the sale of low-fat and fat-free foods. These foods were low in fat, but high in processed carbs—refined starch and sugar—and the obesity epidemic was on. Fast foods came along at the same time. Soft drinks, hamburger buns, pizza pie—these are all packed with processed carbs. These foods also happen to be highly addictive (see chapter 1), which further contributed to the rapid increase in consumption.

Why did the switch to processed carbs lead to the obesity epidemic? For one simple reason: calories from processed carbs are absorbed into the body very quickly, and the quicker such calories come in, the more likely they are to be turned into fat. To understand how this happens, here's some carb-chemistry.

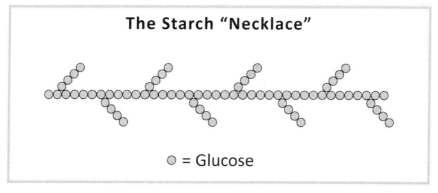

Figure 6. Starch is made up of glucose (sugar) beads strung together in long chains.

Starch is made up of long chains of glucose particles. Glucose is a type of sugar. It is accurate to say that starch is a necklace made from glucose beads. During digestion, the starch necklace is broken up into single glucose beads, which are then absorbed into the body. When you eat starch, you absorb glucose.

As starch is digested and glucose begins to enter the body, it goes down any of three different roads. Some of it is used to make energy, some is put into short-term storage, and some is turned into fat.

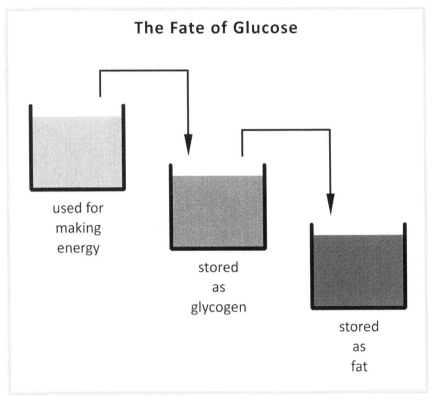

Figure 7. How glucose is used or stored.

How much glucose is used for making energy? Depending on the body size, most of us use between 1,500 to 2,500 calories of energy every twenty-four hours, or between 60 and 105 calories per hour. Let's just use a nice round number—one hundred calories/hour. So, if glucose is coming in at a rate of less than one hundred calories/hour, most of it is likely to be used for making energy. (Note: the body uses both fat and glucose as a fuel source. To keep things simple, I have ignored fat calories in this discussion.)

But if more than one hundred calories worth of glucose comes in during an hour, the excess will be diverted into making a storage form of glucose called glycogen. Glycogen can easily be converted back into glucose when necessary. Glucose stored as glycogen is like having money in a checking account that can be easily withdrawn by writing a check or swiping a debit card. To our distant ancestors, more food was available on some days than on others. The ability to store glucose as glycogen was very useful—on good eating days they deposited excess glucose into this "glycogen checking account" and on days when the pickings were slim, they withdrew some of the glucose and used it for making energy.

Now we have plenty of food all the time. Most of us eat two or three meals daily, often with a snack or two in between. We still occasionally tap into the glycogen account—for example, in the early morning hours after a long night's sleep—but today we have a lot more opportunities to store glucose than we have reasons to take glucose out. And therein lies a problem—the glycogen account can hold only about 1,800 calories of glucose, and because of frequent deposits, the account stays pretty full most the time. It does not take much extra glucose to make the glycogen account max out.

The body has to do something else with the rest of the glucose, and it turns it into fat. Stored fat is like our long-term savings—mutual funds, stocks and bonds, retirement accounts, gold, real estate. Fat is money put aside for future needs. You really don't want to spend your long-term savings unless you absolutely have to. It is the same with the body; it is reluctant to give up the stored fat unless it is forced to.

Unlike the glycogen account, the "fat account" has no upper limit, as many of us know from personal experience. Calories can drip in year after year and the pounds just keep adding up.

It's also a one-way street—unlike the situation with glycogen, the body has no mechanism for turning fat back into glucose. Stored fat has to go down a different road if it is to be used for making energy. This road has many checkpoints (after all, the body doesn't really want to spend its savings), which is why getting rid of fat is not so easy.

To summarize, if carb calories from starch or sugar are coming in slowly, most are likely to be used for making energy. If they are coming in at a faster pace, the excess calories are stored—some as glycogen, and the rest as fat.

So how do you make sure carb calories come in slowly? Simple—by eating natural food.

Starch, sugar, and fiber all come from plants. Almost without exception, every part of every plant contains fiber; fiber

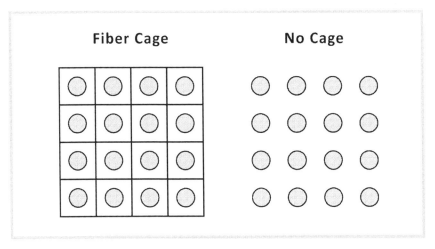

Figure 8. In natural, unprocessed plant products, starch is surrounded by a "fiber cage" that slows down the digestion of starch. Glucose enters the body in a trickle. Processed plant foods usually have no fiber cage. The starch is digested very quickly and glucose floods into the body.

runs through every leaf, root, stem, and fruit. Fiber is the crunch in fruits and veggies. Fiber is also the outer hard shell, or bran, of grains, beans, and other seeds; the fiber shell is what pops when a corn kernel becomes popcorn.

The starch or sugar in plants is surrounded by this fiber. Think of these carbs as being in a "fiber cage." We have to break through this cage before we can get to the carbs. We start this process by chewing the food, and the breaking down of the cage continues in the stomach and intestines. Breaking the cage takes time, so the starch or sugar is freed from the cage slowly and glucose is absorbed into the body just a little bit at a time.

There are actually two kinds of fiber. The fiber we have been talking about so far—the crunchy fiber—is called insoluble fiber because it does not dissolve in water. In addition, beans, lentils, and some fruits such as apples, pears, and bananas contain a second kind of fiber known as soluble fiber. When mixed with water, soluble fiber swells up to form a sticky, invisible sponge. This sponge soaks up glucose; as a result, the absorption of glucose is slowed down even more.

So if we eat any part of a plant that is in its natural state, the presence of one or both kinds of fiber will ensure that any sugar or starch is absorbed slowly, which means it is less likely to be turned into fat.

But if the cage is softened or destroyed before the food is eaten, the carbs will be digested quickly and more of the carb calories will be turned into fat. Cooking softens the cage—the more a food is cooked, the less the crunch and the faster the digestion of any starch or sugar in the food.

But there is something that is even worse than cooking, and that is the processing of plant products. Much of the grain we eat today has been finely ground. Fine grinding completely destroys the cage; it turns the bran—the fiber—into powder. So even when the label says whole grain, the starch is not in a cage. All-purpose or enriched flour is even worse, because the fiber is not only ground into a fine dust; it is also separated and discarded.

Similarly, when an apple is turned into apple juice, the skin and pulp, which contain the fiber, are thrown away and all that is left is cage-free sugar. When we make table sugar from sugarcane or beets, the same thing happens—we throw away the fiber and keep just the sugar. High-fructose corn syrup, of course, also has no fiber.

Eating any glucose-containing food in which the fiber cage is absent or has been destroyed will greatly speed up its digestion, which means glucose will rush into the body, which means more of it will be turned into fat. *That is the big secret.*

That also brings us to the glycemic index.

The Glycemic Index

The glycemic index or the GI of a food that contains starch or glucose tells us how quickly the glucose from that food is absorbed into the body, and its effect on the blood sugar level. Understanding the glycemic index is very helpful for successful weight management.

As glucose is absorbed into the blood from the intestine, the blood glucose level begins to rise. How much it rises, and how long it stays up, depends on the amount of glucose in the food and the speed at which it is entering the body. If the glucose from a meal trickles into the blood a little at a time, the blood glucose level will go up only a little and will come back down quickly. If all the glucose in the meal rushes into the blood at once, the blood glucose level will rise faster, go higher, and take longer to come down.

The effect of a measured amount of food on the blood glucose level is used to calculate its glycemic index. The GI of glucose is arbitrarily set at one hundred and used as the standard. If a food has a GI of 55 or less, it is considered low-glycemic (or low GI); 56-69 is medium GI, and 70 or more is high GI. Beans, lentils, and green veggies have a low GI; most whole grains, long-grain rice (such as basmati rice), pasta, fruits, and starchy veggies have a medium GI; cooked mealy potatoes, short-grain rice, and refined flour such as all-purpose, enriched, and baking flour have a high GI. The higher the GI of a food, the more likely some of the glucose in it will end up as fat.

Of course, we rarely eat any food just by itself. It is more common to eat two or three different foods in one meal. Each of these foods can affect the GI of the meal as a whole. Short-grain white rice has a high GI, but if it is eaten with beans, the GI of the meal goes down because the beans contribute both insoluble and soluble fiber. So, the more correct statement is: The higher the GI of a meal is as a whole, the more likely some of the glucose in it will end up as fat.

If you choose low and medium GI foods, you will prevent most of those food calories from turning into fat. You do control where the calories go.

Glycemic Index vs. Glycemic Load

In addition to the GI of a meal, the portion size also determines how much fat is produced. White bread has a high GI of 70, but if you only eat only one bite, the effect on the blood glucose level will be negligible and none of the glucose is likely to be turned into fat. Conversely, if you eat a whole lot of a lower GI food, the odds are that some of the glucose will end up as fat. The total amount of starch or sugar in a meal determines its glycemic load, or GL. A high glycemic load will encourage the formation of fat.

The program in this book encourages low or medium GI meals in *moderate* portions. If the portion size is moderate, the GI provides all the information you need. You do not have to worry about the GL.

Doctor Alok says:

- Starch is a necklace of glucose beads. During digestion, starch is broken down into glucose, which is then absorbed into the body.
- In the body, glucose can used to make energy, stored as glycogen, or turned into fat.
- The faster glucose is absorbed, the more likely it is that some of it will be turned into fat.

- The starch and sugar in natural plant products such as fruits, roots, leaves, and seeds is surrounded by a fiber cage that slows down digestion and absorption, so the glucose from natural plant products is less likely to be turned into fat.
- Processed foods, such as finely ground grain, sugar, and fruit juice have no fiber cage. The glucose from such foods is absorbed very quickly and is much more likely to be turned into fat.

Chapter 10

Secret #3: Filling Your Stomach Without Filling Your Plate

It is not how much you eat that matters; it's the time you take to eat it in.

Remember the hunger hormone ghrelin from chapter 4? The empty stomach makes ghrelin. Ghrelin gets into the blood, goes to the brain, and tells it to make you hungry. Once you start eating and food begins to enter the stomach, the job of ghrelin is done. Ghrelin production slows down, and within fifteen or twenty minutes after the start of a meal, ghrelin begins to disappear from the blood. As the ghrelin disappears, so does hunger.

About twenty minutes after you start eating your hunger will be gone. Note that the stomach does not have to be full for this to happen. Eat just a moderate amount or eat a lot, it makes little difference. Either way, your hunger will be gone in about twenty minutes.

Once you start eating, something else also happens that reduces hunger. Within twenty to thirty minutes following the start of a meal (faster for liquids, slower for solids), food begins to move from the stomach into the first part of small intestine, the duodenum. When the duodenum sees food, it begins to make hormones that create a sense of satiety, or fullness.

If you eat slowly, your body keeps up with your food intake and turns the hunger switch off at the right time. If you eat too quickly, the body's response lags behind, and by the time your hunger is gone, you have eaten too much. Your stomach is uncomfortably full, and you are likely to make a deposit into your fat account in the next few hours.

This is the moral of the story: If you put a moderate amount of food on your plate and eat it slowly, by about twenty minutes your hunger will be gone. You will be able to push back from the table feeling satisfied. However, if you pile your plate with food and shovel it all down in ten minutes, your stomach will be full, but you will continue to be hungry because there is still a lot of hunger hormone in your system. If a second helping is available, you will take it. You will overeat.

As hunter-gatherers, we ate natural plant food that was rich in fiber. Every bite had to be thoroughly chewed before it could be swallowed. Chewing takes time, so food entered the stomach slowly. The body was able to keep up, and by the time the stomach was full the hunger was gone.

Now we have soft, processed, fiber-free food that needs only minimal chewing—white bread, mashed potatoes, rice; cakes, donuts, and ice cream. Much of today's food requires little chewing, so it goes into the stomach at a fast clip. Even worse, we can just gulp down calories as fruit juice or sugared soda. The stomach overfills because there is no time for the ghrelin to go down and the brain to catch up. It's like a car that is going so fast it runs past the red light before it can stop.

So the secret to eating your fill without filling your plate is to eat slowly. As often as possible, make eating a social activity. Eat with family and friends. Talk a little, eat a little, then talk some more. You'll eat slower and let the process work the way nature intended.

If eating alone, learn to chew the food thoroughly, savoring every bite and experiencing every flavor. Eat for three or four minutes, and when the edge is off your hunger, stop for a minute or two. Put down your knife and fork; read the paper, look around, plan the rest of your day. Start eating again, and after a few minutes, stop once more.

Two or three pauses will add the needed minutes to your meal. You will eat less and feel satisfied. If you just cannot eat slowly, wait fifteen to twenty minutes before you take a second helping. Most of the time, you will find you don't need that second helping after all.

Doctor Alok says:

- The empty stomach makes a hunger hormone called ghrelin. Once food begins to enter the stomach, it begins to make less and less ghrelin—but it takes about twenty minutes for hunger to completely disappear.
- If you put a moderate amount of food on your plate and eat slowly, you will not need a second helping—by the time you finish eating your first serving, your hunger will be gone.

- If you pile your plate high with food and eat it quickly, you will want a second helping even though your stomach is full, because enough time has not gone by for hunger to subside.

Chapter 11

Secret #4: Techniques for Taming Temptation

Perhaps the most common reason for not being able to stick to a healthy eating program is the fact that we are surrounded by artificial, highly tasty and highly addictive designer food—the tiger from chapter 1.

The eating program in the next part of this book will quickly get you de-addicted. But that is just the first step; the bigger problem is avoiding re-addiction. The road to healthy eating is lined with temptation. In today's food environment every meal offers a chance to eat the wrong foods. The tiger is never far away. It waits patiently at the donut shop, the restaurant, the supermarket, the fast-food joint, and even in your own house.

You can't expel the tiger from those other places, but you can certainly banish it from your house. Go through your refrigerator and pantry. Remove anything that might make you lose control. Ice cream, cakes, and pies are no-brainers, but don't forget the honey, the Halloween candy from last year, the brown sugar you love to dump on your cereal—and the box of sweetened cereal too! Chips, salted nuts, raisins, jams, jellies—they all need to go. You can have these foods on "free-styling" days (more on this in chapters 15 and 24), but you cannot have them in your house. They will keep calling to you, and sooner or later you will heed their call.

How about your place of work? How often do you walk into the break room to find half a cake or an open box of donuts on the counter? If you have any influence with your co-workers, use it. Tell them what you are trying to do and enlist their help. Ask them not to tempt you. Even better, talk them into buying this book.

Of course, in spite of your best efforts you will occasionally be ambushed. You are at a restaurant with your friends, and while everyone else is ordering calorie-laden starch-and-fat bombs, you choose to have a nice salad and are feeling really good about your decision. But after you have eaten, the waiter walks up with the dessert tray. You see the tiramisu, the key-lime pie, the cheesecake, and the chocolate mousse. You feel the pull of temptation, the burst of intense desire that turns you into a mindless zombie. You open your mouth to order dessert...

STOP! Point at the tray and say five times: "That is the tiger—*but I am stronger.*" "That is the tiger—*but I am stronger.*" "That is the tiger—*but I am stronger.*" "That is the tiger—*but I am stronger.*" "That is the tiger—*BUT I AM STRONGER.*" This is your mantra. With each repetition you find your resolve hardening, and by the fifth repetition you will be able to say firmly, "Not for me, thank you!" And as you speak these words, you will be overcome with joy. You have once again successfully beaten back the tiger.

You can take pride in winning this battle, but the war will go on. The good news is that as long as you stay de-addicted, you will rarely have any cravings and keeping the tiger at bay is not hard. The bad news is that the tiger never gives up. It shows up many times a day; it rubs against your leg, purring all the while. One moment of weakness and it will have you in its jaws once again.

Before you enter a situation where you might be tempted— a birthday party at work, an evening out with friends—stop for a moment. Gather your defenses; prepare to be strong. Remind yourself that you will be facing the tiger. Then go ahead with your resolve firmed up and your head held high. You will do just fine because it is worth the effort it takes to reach your goal.

Doctor Alok says:

- Beware of the tiger!
- Remove addictive foods from your refrigerator and pantry (and the break room at work, if you can).
- If you are unexpectedly confronted by the tiger, step back, take a deep breath, compose yourself, and stare the tiger down. Each battle won will give you strength for the next one.

Chapter 12

Secret #5: Hunger is the Enemy of Weight Loss

Hunger leads to bad food choices. For successful long-term weight loss, you have to anticipate and avoid hunger.

In most people's minds, trying to lose weight also means going hungry. This is the wrong approach. The hungrier you are, the more tempting everything looks, and the combination of hunger and temptation will take you down the wrong road every time. It seems counterintuitive, but *hunger is the enemy of weight loss.*

There is another reason for avoiding hunger. Scientific studies have shown the body reacts to weight loss by slowing down the metabolism. It's as if the body is trying to protect its fat stores by "pinching its pennies," by using fewer calories to live on.

We don't yet know whether constant hunger pangs in a person who is losing weight add to body's concerns and make it even more determined to fight the weight loss, but anecdotal observations from our weight-management program suggest this might be the case. It is not unusual to see weight loss slow down or stop in individuals who begin to skimp on their meals in an effort to lose weight even faster. While a sensible change in the diet is necessary for weight loss, depriving yourself until you are constantly hungry is counterproductive.

Luckily, avoiding hunger is easy. Weight loss secret #3 showed you how eating even a little bit of food makes hunger go away in about twenty minutes. The secret to avoiding hunger is to eat often, including eating between meals. I remember my grandmother scolding me when I was a kid, "Don't eat between meals—you will lose your appetite!" She was right.

While having a timely breakfast, lunch, and dinner is important, this alone is not enough. Many of us get hungry before it is time to eat the next meal. Breakfast at 7:30 in the morning might be followed by the first stirrings of hunger at 10 or 11 a.m. At first this hunger comes and goes, but by lunchtime it is hard to ignore—and then hunger leads to bad food choices.

The same thing happens between lunch and dinner. It is not unusual for hunger to reappear by about 5 p.m. (the "drive-home" hunger). This hunger makes it hard to get home without succumbing to temptation—it is so easy to pick up a pizza for dinner! Even if you do make it home without straying, you are likely to open the refrigerator door as soon as you walk into the house, and you know what happens next.

But you don't have to lose control. All you need is a snack between breakfast and lunch and another between lunch and dinner.

A small snack, such as twenty almonds or walnut halves and a bit of fruit or cheese will work wonders. You will learn how to make a snack-pack in chapter 19. If you feel even the slightest hunger between breakfast and lunch, eat a few bites. This will get you to lunchtime with no hunger at all, and no hunger means good food choices.

The same strategy can be used in the evening. If you eat a little something up to two hours before dinner, you will stay in control at dinnertime. This can be leftover food in the morning snack-pack that you munch on your drive home, or you can eat a piece of fruit with a few nuts or a small piece of cheese as soon as you walk into the house. Then check the mail, pay the bills, file the credit-card statements, change your clothes – anything to delay eating dinner by about twenty minutes. Now you can walk into the kitchen with the edge already off your hunger.

So here's your eating plan: have breakfast, a small mid-morning snack, lunch, a pre-dinner snack, and dinner, and you will eliminate hunger. The eating program in the next part of the book will make you an expert in each of these steps. By eating often you will eat less, make better food choices, and be less likely to yield to temptation. You will have a slow and steady weight loss, and you will keep off the weight.

Doctor Alok says:

- Hunger leads to bad food choices.
- Having a small, sensible snack between breakfast and lunch, and another snack between lunch and dinner will help you approach mealtimes with no hunger.
- If you are not hungry at lunch and dinner, you are less likely to make bad food choices.

Chapter 13

Secret #6: One Plate Full of Food, One Plate Full of Color = One Life Full of Health

To keep your car running smoothly for a year, you just need to keep filling up the gas tank. But to run smoothly for ten years, your car needs more than fill-ups. It also needs tune-ups—an oil change once in a while, new belts, new sparkplugs. If your sparkplugs are dirty, it doesn't matter how much gas you put in your tank—you aren't going anywhere.

The body works the same way. For a long and healthy life, it needs both fill-ups and tune-ups. So, of the two major daily meals—lunch and dinner—one should be a "fill-up" meal and the other a "tune-up" meal.

Carbohydrates, fat, and protein are fill-up foods. We use carbohydrates and fat for making energy, and protein for keeping our muscles and organs in good repair.

But just having fill-up foods is not enough. We also need tune-up foods such as vitamins and minerals and anti-oxidants and omega-3 fatty acids. Vitamins and minerals keep the metabolism running smoothly. Anti-oxidants detoxify oxygen radicals, or "free radicals," that are a by-product of making energy.

Omega-3 fatty acids, which are found not only in marine algae and fish but also in the green parts of plants, help to keep the body's inflammatory reactions in check and the blood from clotting too readily.

We need tune-up foods in small amounts, but we do need them. Sailors suffered and died from scurvy for hundreds of years for the lack of a little lime juice to give them vitamin C. Up to half a million children worldwide still go blind every year from a deficiency of vitamin A. Even in a developed country such as the United States, a teenager's fast-food diet probably does not have enough anti-oxidants and omega-3 fatty acids.

A simple but effective way to make sure we are getting both fill-up foods and tune-up foods is to plan one major meal every day as a fill-up meal and the other as a tune-up meal. However, to complete the food picture, we need one more vital ingredient: fiber.

Strictly speaking, fiber is neither a fill-up nor a tune-up food because humans do not have the ability to digest and absorb fiber. Fiber just makes other foods more healthy (see secret #2). Fiber also prevents constipation and thus lowers the risk of appendicitis, diverticulosis, and perhaps even colon cancer. So both the fill-up meal and the tune-up meal should contain some fiber.

What do the fill-up and tune-up meals look like?

The Fill-Up Meal

This is the sustenance meal. The goal is to provide a healthy amount of carbs, protein, and fat, along with some natural fiber from vegetables and/or fruits. A good way of putting together a sustenance meal is to imagine a dinner plate divided into three equal parts as shown below.

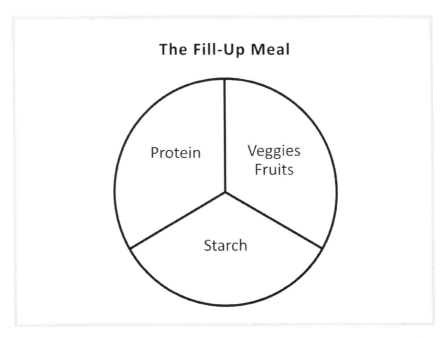

Figure 9. The fill-up meal. Don't load the food all the way to the edge of the plate. Leave a little empty space around the edges.

The protein is in one third-of the plate, the starch (carbohydrates) is in the next third, and the vegetables/fruits are in the last third. If using a full-size dinner plate, leave a one-inch margin clear around the edges of the plate. In reality, colorful veggies need not be restricted to a third of a plate, but the protein and starch should stay within their boundaries. Note that root vegetables count as starch, not veggies. Of course, not every meal has to be arranged like this, but this gives you an idea of how much of each type of food should be contained in a sustenance meal.

Leaner cuts of beef, skinless poultry, baked or broiled fish, beans, and tofu are all good protein choices. The meats should not be high in saturated fat. Substituting grass-fed beef, free-range chicken, or ocean fish (more omega-3) when possible is even better but not essential. The veggies should be left a little crunchy to preserve the fiber cage (see chapter 9).

The choice of starch, or carbohydrate, depends on your situation. If you are not trying to lose weight, you can use any carbohydrate, free or caged. Bread, potatoes, white rice, pasta—it does not matter because you are limiting the amount to a third of the plate. However, if you are trying to lose weight, use low GI carbohydrates that have at least some fiber. Long-grain brown rice, quinoa, whole-wheat pasta, sprouted grain or whole-grain bread, and beans are all good. Note that beans can be used both as a protein and as a carb—they have both, along with a good amount of fiber.

Eat your fill-up meal slowly, taking about twenty minutes. This is critical! Eating slowly gives the body a chance to keep up with the food intake so it can adjust the hunger accordingly. If at the end of twenty minutes you are still hungry, eat some more. But if you follow the twenty-minute rule, odds are you will not need a second helping.

The Tune-Up Meal

The goal of the tune-up meal is to get lots of anti-oxidants, vitamins, and minerals along with natural plant fiber and omega-3 fatty acids. *Two-thirds or more of the tune-up meal should consist of colorful and crunchy vegetables and fruits.* The color provides anti-oxidants, vitamins, minerals, and some omega-3; the crunch is the fiber.

A multi-colored salad is an excellent tune-up meal. In addition to vegetables and fruits, your salad should also have some protein and a little fat, otherwise you risk being hungry again in an hour or two. Put some chicken or fish, beans, and/or cheese on the plate. Meat, fish, or cheese will provide protein and fat; beans are a good source of protein and fiber. However, as mentioned above, the veggies and fruits should clearly be the stars of the show, constituting two-thirds or more of the meal.

A tune-up meal need not always be raw. Veggies can be grilled, broiled, sautéed lightly, or steamed as long as they retain their color and some of the crunch, meaning the natural goodness has not been cooked out.

There should be no fiber-free starch and sugar in the tune-up meal. If you are eating in a restaurant, send back the garlic bread, the pita, the rolls, or the chips.

So there it is. A plate full of food (the fill-up meal) and a plate full of color (the tune-up meal) each day will ensure your body has everything it needs. This simple eating regimen will improve your health, help you lose weight, and keep you brimming with energy.

Doctor Alok says:

- One major daily meal should be a fill-up, or sustenance, meal—meat, vegetables, and carbs in moderate amounts, eaten slowly to give the hunger hormone a chance to go down.
- The other major daily meal should be a tune-up meal, full of colorful leaves, vegetables, and fruits that are brimming with vitamins, fiber, and anti-oxidants.

Chapter 14

Secret #7: You Can't Sweat Out the Fat

Moderate exercise, such as a brisk thirty-minute walk three or four days a week is an important part of a healthy lifestyle. In fact, as people get older and their metabolism begins to slow down, moderate exercise can be helpful in jump-starting and maintaining weight loss. But be careful of doing too much, because excessive exercise can interfere with weight loss. There are at least two reasons for this.

The first is that exercising can become an excuse for eating the wrong things. You run three miles, then stop by the coffee shop and have the café mocha because you have "earned" it. By running three miles you have used up about three hundred calories, but a medium-sized café mocha has three hundred and sixty calories. Most impulse food contains more calories than you might suspect. You will need to run five miles to make up for eating a Big Mac—and that's without the fries.

There is a second reason. In some people, exercise tends to increase hunger. If you are on a healthy eating regimen and losing weight, and then start an exercise program, you need to watch your body's response carefully. If you find you are so hungry when you come home from the gym that you cannot stick to your healthy eating regimen, exercise is not a good weight-loss tool for you. Cut back on the exercise. Of course if you find that you can exercise, continue to stay on your eating program, and keep losing weight—go for it.

Doctor Alok says:

- Moderate exercise is part of a healthy lifestyle, but too much exercise can interfere with weight loss because-
- Exercising gives us the permission to eat the wrong things, and
- In some people, too much exercise can increase hunger and make it harder to stick to a healthy eating regimen.

Chapter 15

Secret #8: Cheating Occasionally is Good for Weight Loss

We won't call it cheating, though—let's call it freestyling instead. Eating something off-program a couple of times a week, a food item or two that will give you pleasure without making you lose control, is good practice. It gives you something to look forward to and makes it easier to stay on the program.

But there is more. Even though there are no scientific studies (as yet) to back this up, experience in our program suggests that an occasional larger-than-usual meal helps to keep the weight loss going and delays the first plateau. In fact, people even report breaking through a plateau right after a freestyling meal. It's as if the body is reassured there is not a scarcity of food, so it stops fighting the weight loss.

There is a lot more on freestyling in chapter 24.

Doctor Alok says:

- Occasional, controlled cheating is good for weight loss.

Part 4:

Getting Started—The First Two Weeks

An Overview

It's time to start losing weight. The first two weeks will launch you into the program. These are your training weeks, a time to quickly learn some new skills.

The shopping lists, daily menus, and recipes will guide you every step of the way. You will learn to prepare simple but tasty low-glycemic food. Planning ahead, putting together snack-packs, having a tune-up and a fill-up meal daily—it's all there. At the end of two weeks you will be able to say, "I know how to do this!" You will also realize you are putting into practice the secrets from the previous section.

The biggest change you are likely to notice in the first few days of the program is that your cravings are gone. You have become de-addicted to designer foods. This de-addiction usually happens within two to five days, but sometimes it takes a little longer, so stick with it. Make sure you eat every meal and snack at the prescribed times because this will help you fight the cravings.

Even after the cravings have disappeared, you will occasionally feel hungry. This is normal hunger. Your body is used to a certain food intake and is making you aware that you are falling short. This hunger will also gradually subside.

During these first two weeks, you will eat colorful vegetables and a small amount of fruit, beans and meat, medium and low GI carbohydrates, and some fat. The food will be lightly seasoned without an excess of spices and no sugar or sugar substitutes because these can keep the addictive hunger going. Also, there is no freestyling or dessert in the first two weeks.

You will not be eating high GI carbohydrates, so your blood sugar level will stabilize. You will have more energy and the afternoon low will be a thing of the past. You will sleep better at night and wake up feeling refreshed.

Note: If you are taking medication for diabetes, high blood pressure, or anything else, you need to monitor yourself carefully. *The dose of medications might need to be reduced even before you start losing weight.* Keep in touch with your doctor.

Chapter 16

Six Steps that
Lead to Success

The first few days of the program are hard because you are making a sharp U-turn in *what* you eat, *when* you eat, and *how* you eat. Here are some pointers to help you along.

1. To avoid temptation, it is best to clear your refrigerator and pantry of any forbidden foods. Get rid of anything that might call out to you. Shoo those tigers out!

Ice cream and other frozen treats, cakes and pies, cookies and candy, salted nuts and bags of potato or corn chips—these are no-brainers, but don't forget the sugared cereal, the bottle of honey or agave nectar, the heavy cream, raisins and sweetened cranberries, brown sugar, and for now, even juicy fruits such as grapes and watermelon. Any food that can make you slip should be out of the house. You might also want to review weight-loss secret #4—Techniques for Taming Temptation.

2. Follow the program as closely as you can. Read the shopping lists, menus, and recipes and stick to them. If you have an allergy or a strong dislike for a food—or some other valid reason for not eating a particular food item—you can substitute the same meal from a different day, such as a breakfast for a

breakfast or a lunch for a lunch. But do not try to be inventive, do not cut corners, do not push the envelope.

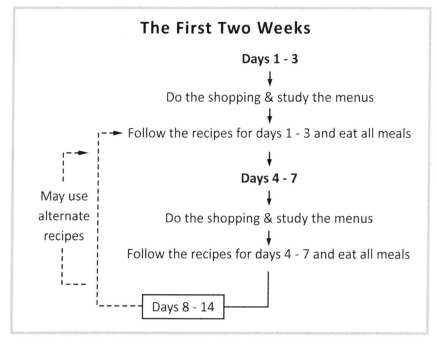

Figure 10. The first two weeks. See the text for details.

The first week is divided into a three-day and a four-day period, with a shopping list for each of the two periods. There is a menu for each day and a recipe for every item on the menu. To keep the shopping list manageable, many of the menu items are repeated from day to day. The recipes you use in the first and second weeks are important educational tools. After the two weeks are over, they will become the foundations for your own recipes.

Each day's menu lists the breakfast, a morning snack, the tune-up meal, the pre-dinner snack, and the fill-up meal. The second week is a repetition of the first, except that you can start using recipes from the alternate recipes section in chapter 22 so you don't have to eat the same things over and over again.

3. Move meals around if you need to. There is no taboo against having the fill-up meal for lunch and the tune-up meal at dinnertime. But you cannot add or subtract a meal—you must have breakfast, the morning snack, lunch, the pre-dinner snack, and dinner (in that order) every day.

4. Plan ahead! You must make time every day to study the menu for the next day. Make sure you have all necessary ingredients on hand. If you need to prepare and pack food to take with you the next day, go ahead and do so. Consider leaving your car keys in the refrigerator on the packet of food as a reminder to take the packet with you.

5. Eat slowly. Take fifteen to twenty minutes to finish lunch and dinner. If it has been at least twenty minutes since you started eating and you are still hungry, eat some more—but the need for a second helping should be the exception, not the rule. Also, make sure the second helping is for hunger and not desire.

6. Keep a note of your daily weight. Weigh yourself at the same time every day, preferably in the morning.

Note: This two-week program is not designed for vigorous exercise. Moderate exercise such as a brisk walk three or four times a week is fine.

Chapter 17

Before You Start:
Finding the Right Fit

If your BMI is less than 25, you are already in good shape. Review and understand this section, but you do not need to strictly follow the program. Once you are familiar with the basics—the types of food, simple food preparation without excess salt or spices, the five daily meals—you can go directly to the Part V, "Hanging Tough—The Next Six Months."

If your BMI is 25 or higher, go to "Day 1."

Day 1

You should have already finished your shopping before starting the program on this first day. Follow the daily menus and recipes *exactly as written*. The only exceptions are food allergies, a really strong dislike for a food, or another valid reason for not eating a food item. If this is so, you can make substitutions as discussed in chapter 16. Remember to eat slowly, especially the fill-up meal. Expect some hunger and cravings for the first few days. Be strong, and enjoy the weight loss.

Do not be frustrated by the time it takes to put your meals together. You will become better at this with every passing day.

Read ahead to end of the book, then start at the beginning and read this book a second time. The more familiar you become with the contents, the greater are your odds of success.

Day 8

This is the beginning of your second week. If your starting BMI was between 25 and 29, take stock. Are you well-settled into the program and don't have excessive hunger? Then continue into the second week. However, if you find you are beginning to get hungry again towards the end of the first week, you can go directly to day fifteen. You have less excess fat and less weight to lose than those with a higher BMI, and your body may begin to protest the rapid weight loss after the first week by increasing your hunger. This is not addictive hunger; it is increased normal hunger (see chapter 4). But if hunger is not a problem, by all means continue into the second week of the program.

If your starting BMI was 30 or higher, definitely do the second week of the program. Remember that you are now allowed to use recipes from the alternate recipes section (chapter 22).

Life after the first two weeks is covered in Part V, "Hanging Tough—The Next Six Months."

Chapter 18

The Big Day:
On Your Mark, Set, Go!

Find a two-week block of time without a vacation or long business trip and go for it. Pick a date and *start*. Don't let your excitement and energy drain away. *You can do it!*

Don't keep looking for the perfect moment to start; there never will be one. Don't keep waiting for a two-week block that is free of weddings and parties, or when the kids are in (or out of) school, or when a high-stress project at work is done. Life happens. Deal with it. Just pick a date, do your shopping, and start.

If you have a job with a five-day work week, starting on a Monday makes it easier to slide into the program. Your day is more structured and being at work is a useful distraction from food cravings. Do your shopping and food preparation over the weekend so you can start with breakfast on Monday morning. If you don't work outside the home, it does not matter which day you start. *Either way, make sure you have removed all temptation from the refrigerator and pantry*—see chapter 16.

Short business trips within the first two weeks are okay; just pack food to take with you. If you are driving, take a cooler full of food; if you are flying, pack your food. Call the hotel and ask for a refrigerator and a microwave in your room. Most hotels will oblige you even if those are not standard appliances for the room.

You will be quite busy for the first few days—shopping and chopping, cooking and packing. Do not be discouraged because you are learning to give structure to your eating. You are eating healthy in a world that is eating unhealthy—of course it's hard work. It's like renting a car in a country in which everyone drives on the left instead of the right. The first few days are stressful. But soon driving becomes less of a strain. You start to look around and take in the scenery. The tension is gone. You begin to enjoy yourself.

It is the same with this program. With every passing day, shopping, cooking, and packing will take less and less time. As your weight goes down, your enthusiasm and energy level will go up. Above all, you will have a deep sense of satisfaction because you now control your food instead of your food controlling you.

Weight Loss in the First Two Weeks

Most people lose between five and twelve pounds in the first two weeks. But everyone is different. If you faithfully follow the plan but lose fewer than five pounds, don't worry about it. Your body may not be ready to start giving up its fat. Be patient, stay on the program, and you will lose weight. Also, if you have already been losing weight when you start the program your initial weight loss may be less.

Remember that losing weight becomes more difficult as we get older. If you are over sixty, it might take a while to kick-start the weight loss. Another consideration is the starting BMI; if this was less than thirty, you may lose less weight in the first two weeks simply because there is less to lose. Also, if you are carrying most of your weight in your hips and thighs and only a little around the waist, you may lose weight more slowly. And ladies—remember that men generally lose weight faster than women.

Don't compare yourself to others. Patience is the key. Stay on the program and do not attempt to force the weight loss by eating even less—this might make the body fight back harder.

Chapter 19

Shopping List and
Menus for Days 1-3

Shopping List: Per Person

Produce

3 small apples

1 pint (lb.) fresh strawberries

1 lemon

1 head of broccoli

1 zucchini

1 avocado

1 package mushrooms (for kabobs and breadless burger)

1 small container alfalfa sprouts (if desired, for burger)

2 English (or regular) cucumbers

2 bags salad greens of choice

1 head bok choy

2 fresh carrots

1 bunch of green onions

3 bell peppers (any color)

3 tomatoes plus 1 pkg. cherry tomatoes (for kabobs)

2 onions (1 purple, 1 yellow or white)

1 head of garlic

Baked Goods/Frozen Foods

1 loaf sprouted grain bread (such as Ezekiel bread in the orange wrapper) in the frozen food section
1 package sprouted grain/whole grain/low carb tortillas (if low carb are not available, get whole grain, fresh, not frozen)
1 package sprouted grain/whole grain/low carb pita pocket bread. If pita pocket bread is not available, use a tortilla as a wrap, or just use a slice of the sprouted grain bread.

Dairy

1 dozen eggs
1 8-oz. pkg. regular (not low-fat) shredded cheddar cheese
1 4-oz. container crumbled feta cheese
1 brick hard, aged cheese (cheddar, Gouda)

Bulk/Canned/Dried

1 8-oz. bag raw unsalted almonds, skin-on
1 15-oz. can garbanzo beans
2 15-oz. cans pinto beans
2 15-oz. cans kidney beans
1 2.5-oz. can black olives, chopped
1 15-oz. can cut green beans
1 15-oz. can cut yellow (wax) beans

Seasonings/Condiments

1 bottle seasoned salt (your preference)
Extra virgin olive oil
1 bottle vinaigrette (oil and vinegar) dressing with no added sugar (or make your own; see recipes in chapter 21 and obtain the ingredients listed in the recipe)

1 jar natural peanut butter (no trans-fat)

1 bottle Dijon mustard

Meat

6 raw chicken breasts (halves)

1 raw or frozen hamburger, turkey, veggie, or buffalo patty (buy a multi-pack and freeze the extra)

Menus

Note: For each item on the menu, use the recipe provided in the recipe section (chapter 21).

Tip: The evening before you start the program (Day 1), season and sauté two of the chicken breast halves and keep them in the refrigerator (see chapter 21 for recipe). You will use these cooked chicken breast halves for lunch for the first two days.

Day 1

Breakfast
Tortilla with scrambled egg and cheese (the cheese is optional)

Morning Snack
½ cubed apple

20 almonds (You don't have to eat all twenty if you are not hungry; you can use the leftover almonds for the evening snack. But if you are hungry, eat them all.)

Tune-up Meal
Lunch salad topped with 1 sliced chicken breast. Eat
your fill of salad.

Pre-dinner Snack
2-3 strawberries or ½ apple
½" X 1" X 2" (1 oz.) piece of hard cheese (or the leftover
almonds from the morning)

Fill-up Meal
Bare Mountain Burger
Pinto beans
Side salad or roasted vegetables

Day 2

Breakfast
Sprouted grain toast with peanut butter and fruit

Morning Snack
½ cubed apple
20 almonds

Tune-up Meal
Lunch salad topped with 1 sliced chicken breast. Eat
your fill of salad.

Pre-dinner Snack

2-3 strawberries or ½ apple

½" X 1" X 2" (1 oz.) piece of hard cheese (or leftover almonds from the morning)

Fill-up Meal

Chicken kabobs

3-bean salad (will be used for two meals)

Side salad or roasted vegetables

Day 3

Breakfast

Toasted ½ pita pocket with scrambled egg and cheese

Morning Snack

½ cubed apple

20 almonds

Tune-up Meal

Chicken Garbanzo Bean salad in ½ pita or tortilla (may prepare the day before and keep)

Veggie strips: cucumber, broccoli, bell pepper, or other (your choice—there is no recipe for this) with vinaigrette dressing. Eat your fill.

Pre-dinner Snack
2-3 strawberries or ½ apple

½" X 1" X 2" (1 oz.) piece of hard cheese (or leftover almonds from the morning)

Fill-up Meal
Chicken kabob

3-bean salad

Side salad or roasted vegetables

*Tip #1: Reserve some of the sautéed chicken for the pre-dinner snack on Day 4

*Tip #2: Reserve the remaining portion of Chicken Garbanzo Bean salad for lunch on Day 4

Chapter 20

Shopping List and Menus for Days 4-7

Shopping list: Per Person

Produce

1 pear

2 apples

1 lime

2 cucumbers

1 bag salad greens of your choice (or fresh salad greens)

1 bag fresh spinach

2 onions (one purple, one yellow or white)

4 medium tomatoes

1 leek (or a bunch of green onions) if the bunch you previously bought is finished

2 bell peppers (any color)

1 pint grape tomatoes

1 cup bean sprouts

Small container of mint leaves

1 head Boston leaf lettuce for wraps and salad (may substitute other large leaf lettuce such as green leaf, Romaine, Red Leaf)

Additional vegetables as desired (see Day 4-7 menu and the recipe section for ideas about using additional vegetables)

Frozen Foods
1 bag frozen, unsalted shelled soy beans (edamame). These are usually found in the frozen vegetables section.

Dairy
Small container of shredded parmesan cheese

Bulk/Canned/Dried
8-oz. cup wild rice (from bulk bins or boxed on the shelf)
8-oz. bag walnut halves
1 small bag (2 tablespoons) sliced almonds (baking aisle or bulk bins)
½ cup unsalted roasted shelled peanuts (optional topping for chicken lettuce wraps)

Meat
2 firm white fish filets (such as red snapper, trout, halibut, flounder)
2 rib loin (or other cut) pork chops
1 skinless, boneless chicken breast half
1 lb. ground turkey or beef (or grass-fed beef)

Menus

Day 4

Breakfast
Scrambled egg frittata

Morning Snack
¼ cup thawed edamame
10 walnut halves

Tune-up Meal
Leftover Chicken Garbanzo Bean Salad in ½ pita pocket
or tortilla wrap
Side salad topped with half an apple, cubed

Pre-dinner Snack
3-4 pieces of chicken (saved from Day 3)
10 walnut halves

Fill-up Meal
Basil fish filet (bake 2 filets; you will use one for lunch
on Day 5)
Wild rice salad (will need 4 servings for use at different
times)
Side salad or roasted vegetables

Day 5

Breakfast:
Sprouted grain toast with peanut butter and apple

Morning Snack
¼ cup thawed edamame
10 walnut halves

Tune-up Meal
Lunch salad topped with fish (use the 3-oz. baked filet from Day 4). Eat your fill of salad.

Pre-dinner Snack
½ cubed apple
10 walnut halves

Fill-up Meal
Pork chop
Wild rice salad
Side salad or roasted vegetables

Day 6

Breakfast
Tortilla with scrambled egg and cheese (the cheese is optional)

Morning Snack
¼ cup thawed edamame
10 walnut halves

Tune-up Meal
Spinach salad topped with pork
Wild rice salad

Pre-dinner Snack
½ cubed apple
10 walnut halves

Fill-up Meal
Turkey chili (save some for next day)
Wild rice salad
Side salad or roasted vegetables

Day 7

Breakfast
Sprouted grain toast topped with thinly sliced boiled egg and sliced cucumber with a dash of salt and pepper

Morning Snack
¼ cup thawed edamame
10 walnut halves or any of the other morning snacks

Tune-up Meal
Chicken lettuce wraps

Pre-dinner snack
½ cubed apple
10 walnut halves

Dinner
Turkey chili
1 slice sprouted grain toast
Roasted vegetables—use any leftover vegetables such as broccoli, zucchini, onion, mushrooms, tomato

Chapter 21

Recipes for the First Two Weeks

Recipes are listed in the approximate order in which they appear on the eating schedule.

Sautéed Chicken Breast
1. To ensure the chicken is completely cooked, slice each chicken breast horizontally in half so there are two pieces of similar thickness.
2. Dust with seasoned salt or salt and pepper.
3. Prepare sauté pan by heating to medium high and adding 1 teaspoon of vegetable oil (canola or other).
4. Add chicken and cook for about five minutes on each side until no longer pink in the middle.
5. Slice into strips or cut into bite-sized pieces and keep in refrigerator for use as salad topping.

Tortilla with scrambled egg and cheese
1. Scramble 1 egg (one additional egg white may be added if desired).
2. Fold half a tortilla and toast in a toaster.

3. Put scrambled egg inside folded-over tortilla.
4. Top with ¼ cup of shredded cheddar cheese, if desired.

Lunch salad with mixed greens, veggies, feta cheese

2-3 cups mixed greens

½ tomato, chopped or sliced

½ cucumber, chopped or sliced

1/3 bell pepper, chopped or sliced

2 tablespoons crumbled feta cheese

Place all ingredients into a bowl and drizzle with approximately 1 tablespoon vinaigrette dressing. Toss to coat.

Vinaigrettes
Basic white wine vinaigrette (makes 1 cup):

¼ cup white wine vinegar

¼ teaspoon salt

1 small clove of garlic, minced

2 teaspoons Dijon mustard

1/8 teaspoon freshly cracked black pepper

¾ cup extra virgin olive oil

1. In a medium bowl, whisk together the vinegar and salt.
2. When the salt has dissolved, add the garlic, mustard, thyme, and pepper and gradually whisk in the olive oil.

Sherry - walnut vinaigrette (makes 1 cup):

¼ cup sherry vinegar

¼ teaspoon sea salt

1/8 teaspoon freshly cracked black pepper

¾ cup walnut (or part safflower or canola) oil

1. In a medium bowl, whisk together vinegar, salt, and pepper.
2. When the salt has dissolved, whisk in the oil. Taste the walnut oil before using—it may need to be combined with a mild-flavored oil so as to not overwhelm the other flavors.

Cilantro-basil vinaigrette (makes 1 cup):

¼ cup white balsamic vinegar

2-3 tablespoons each minced fresh cilantro and basil

¼ teaspoon salt

1/8 teaspoon freshly cracked black pepper

¾ cup extra virgin olive oil

1. In a medium bowl, whisk together vinegar, salt, and pepper.
2. When the salt has dissolved, whisk in the olive oil, cilantro, and basil.

Bare Mountain Burger

This burger is served without a bun, but it is piled high with a variety of vegetables.

1. Cook one hamburger, turkey, veggie, or bison burger patty according to package instructions.
2. Top with vegetables or toppings of your choice such as:

   a. Sliced avocado
   b. ½ cup washed and dried bean sprouts

    c. Roasted red bell pepper

    d. Any amount of any type of leafy greens

    e. Hummus

    f. Sliced tomato

    g. Leeks or green onion

    h. Sliced onion

    i. Sautéed eggplant

    j. Sliced mushrooms

    k. Pickles

    l. Dijon mustard.

3. Serve with a side of pinto beans.

Pinto Beans

1 clove of garlic
½ cup chopped yellow onion
1 15-oz. can pinto beans

1. Heat 1 teaspoon olive oil in sauce pan.
2. Add 1 chopped garlic clove and ½ cup chopped yellow onion. Cook until onion is translucent.
3. Open 1 can of pinto beans and rinse. Add to pan and sauté for 2 minutes or until heated through. One serving = ½ cup.

Side Salad (or may use leftover lunch salad)

¼ cup basic white wine vinaigrette
1 head of fresh bok choy, very thinly sliced
2 medium carrots, shredded

Green onions, thinly sliced

Stir vinaigrette together with the veggies.

Roasted vegetables
1. Use the same vegetables as in the kabob recipe in this chapter and season them in the same manner.
2. Arrange the veggies in a single layer on a rack in a baking dish lined with foil.
3. Place the dish in an oven preheated to 475 degrees.
4. Start checking for doneness at 10-15 minutes. Remove the veggies when the edges begin to char.

Another option:
1. Heat 2 tablespoons of vegetable oil in a large saucepan.
2. When the oil is quite hot (medium to medium high), add the cut veggies.
3. Season with salt, ground black pepper, and any other spices you want to experiment with.
4. Stir vigorously for 5-10 minutes, adding a pinch of salt and seasoning after each stir.
5. Remove the veggies while still crunchy. The broccoli tastes great when the outer portions of the florets are browned but the stems are still firm.

Toast with peanut butter and fruit
1. Toast 1 slice of sprouted grain bread in toaster.
2. Spread with 1 tablespoon peanut butter and layer with ½ sliced apple or 3 sliced strawberries.

Shrimp, Chicken, or Beef Kabobs

Jumbo shrimp, approx. 4-5 shrimp per serving (or 8-10 smaller shrimp per serving)

OR boneless chicken breasts (approx. 1 breast per serving)

OR beef—sirloin steak or other (1 palm size piece of meat per serving)

Any three or more of the following:

Bell pepper, cut into 1-inch squares

Mushrooms, sliced in half lengthwise

Onion, cut into 1- to 2-inch chunks and separated into individual layers

Broccoli (fresh) cut into 1 ½-inch florets

Zucchini, cut into ½-inch slices

Any other firm vegetable

1. Shrimp should be whole, peeled, and cleaned.
2. Chicken and beef should be cut into 1-inch cubes.
3. Sprinkle the meat with seasoned salt and mix everything thoroughly with your hand.
4. Drizzle with olive oil and mix thoroughly again.
5. Cover and let sit in the refrigerator for at least an hour; overnight in the refrigerator is even better.
6. Sprinkle salt and black pepper on the vegetable pieces and drizzle with olive oil; mix.
7. Preheat the oven to 475 degrees F.
8. Skewer the meat and vegetables on separate skewers (the cooking time for each is different).
9. Suspend the skewers across a baking pan. Alternatively, spread meat and vegetables without skewers on a

baking pan lined with aluminum foil. Place the pan in the oven.

The approximate cooking time is as follows:
   a. Mushrooms: 10 minutes
   b. Veggies: 12-15 minutes or until the edges begin to char.
   c. Chicken: 13-15 minutes
   d. Beef: 15-18 minutes, depending on the cut—keep checking!
   e. Jumbo shrimp: 10 minutes (smaller shrimp will take less time)

As each item comes out, slide the pieces off the skewer into a bowl. Toss everything together so some of the vegetable juices coat and flavor the meat. Enjoy!

Simple 3-Bean Salad
1 can (15 to 16 ounces) cut green beans, no added salt
1 can (15 to 16 ounces) cut yellow beans
1 can (15 to 16 ounces) red kidney beans
1/2 bell pepper, chopped
1/4 cup sliced purple onion
1/3 cup vinaigrette dressing
1/2 teaspoon salt
1/2 teaspoon pepper

   1. Rinse and drain the beans.
   2. Combine beans, green pepper, and sliced onion.

3. Pour dressing over bean mixture.
4. Toss well and chill for at least 4 hours. Store in refrigerator.

Chicken Garbanzo Bean Salad

1 cooked chicken breast, shredded or chopped into small pieces
½ bell pepper, diced (any color)
1 can garbanzo beans, rinsed
¼ cup onion, chopped
6 black olives, chopped
1 teaspoon olive oil
1 tablespoon lemon juice
Shredded cheddar cheese
½ pita pocket or 1 tortilla for each serving

1. Combine all ingredients.
2. Pile onto a tortilla and roll it up, or fill ½ toasted pita pocket. Makes 2-3 servings.

Scrambled Egg Frittata

1 egg and 1 egg white
1 cup of pre-washed fresh spinach
½ cup cooked or canned and washed beans (may use leftover pinto beans)
1 leek or 3 green onions
½ cup shredded cheddar cheese

1. Wash and chop the leek (use only the white part and discard the green portion).

2. Whisk the egg and egg white in a bowl.

3. Put the leek into a frying pan lightly coated with cooking spray. Sauté for 2-3 minutes until it softens. (If using green onion, chop and use the green portion and add at the end).

4. Add the beans and spinach and press down with a spatula so that spinach begins to wilt.

5. Pour the egg over the top.

6. Top with the cheese and season with a pinch of salt and freshly ground pepper if desired.

7. Cook for another 3 minutes on low heat. The frittata is done when egg no longer runs and the spinach is wilted.

Basil Fish Filet

2 fish filets, each 4-5 oz.
1 tablespoon dried basil
½ teaspoon black pepper
2 tablespoons parmesan cheese
Cooking spray

1. Cover baking sheet with foil, spray with cooking spray.

2. Cut fish in serving size portions. Place on baking sheet, then spray fish lightly with cooking spray.

3. Combine basil, pepper, and cheese. Sprinkle over fish.

4. Bake at 400 degrees F until done (10-15 min). 1 serving = 1 fish filet.

Wild Rice Salad

1 cup wild rice

3 green onions (scallions)

1 cup grape tomatoes

¼ cup vinaigrette dressing (see recipes provided in this chapter)

1. Cook 1 cup wild rice according to package directions and set aside to cool.
2. Slice the green portion of the scallions thinly.
3. Halve the grape tomatoes.
4. Add ingredients to the rice and mix with dressing. Serve chilled. 1 serving = ¾ cup.

Pork Chops

2 pork chops

¼ teaspoon salt

¼ teaspoon pepper

¼ teaspoon paprika

¼ teaspoon sage

¼ teaspoon thyme

1 tablespoon olive oil

1/2 onion, sliced

1. Preheat oven to 425 degrees F.
2. Mix the dry ingredients and rub into both sides of the pork chops.
3. Brown chops in oil on medium heat for 2-3 minutes on each side.
4. Place each of the chops on a piece of aluminum foil.

5. Layer each with 2-3 thinly sliced onion rings. Make a pouch with the foil and seal tightly.
6. Place on baking sheet and bake for 30 minutes.
7. Reserve the juice from each foil packet and drizzle on the chops.

Spinach Salad Topped with Pork

2 cups washed spinach leaves (see chapter 39 for instructions on how to wash and drain leaves)

¼ red onion, thinly sliced

½ fresh apple or pear, chopped into bite-sized pieces

2 tablespoons thinly sliced almonds

2 tablespoons crumbled cheese such as feta or gorgonzola

1 tablespoon oil and vinegar dressing (citrus vinaigrette works well)

1. Combine all ingredients.
2. Top with half of a pork chop, thinly sliced (see recipe above).

Turkey Chili

1 lb. ground turkey (or grass-fed ground beef or regular ground beef)

¾ medium onion, chopped

1 green bell pepper, diced

2 cloves garlic, minced

2 ripe Roma tomatoes, chopped

1 can (15-oz.) pinto or kidney beans, well-drained and washed

1 tablespoon sun dried tomato paste

1 tablespoon chili powder

½ cup water

Salt to taste

1. In a large nonstick skillet, cook turkey, onion, and garlic over medium heat until turkey loses its pink color.

2. Stir in remaining ingredients; bring to boil. Cover, reduce heat, and simmer 15-20 minutes.

Chicken Lettuce Wraps

1 skinless, boneless chicken breast half

2 Boston lettuce leaves

¼ cup fresh mint leaves

½ cup bean sprouts (store bought or home sprouted mung beans—see recipe in chapter 22)

2 lime wedges

Chopped peanuts (optional)

Other optional vegetables: shredded carrot, sliced cucumber, water chestnuts, bamboo shoots, jicama, bell pepper, shredded cabbage.

1. Slice chicken breast horizontally into two pieces of equal thickness.

2. Heat a large nonstick sauté pan over medium high heat.

3. Coat pan with olive oil.

4. Add chicken to pan; cook for about five minutes on each side until no longer pink in the middle.

5. Let chicken stand 5 minutes before slicing thinly.
6. Divide chicken evenly among lettuce leaves; top each lettuce leaf with mint, sprouts, and other vegetables.
7. Drizzle each open wrap with lime juice.
8. Serve with lime wedges; garnish with chopped peanuts, if desired.

Chapter 22

Alternate Recipes for the Second Week

If you want to try something else during the second week, here are some suggestions.

Breakfast Alternates

Toast Toppers

The breakfast toast slice can be topped with any of the following:

a. Hummus and sliced tomatoes
b. A slice of cheddar cheese, a slice of roasted turkey breast, sliced tomato/spinach/lettuce
c. Hummus and olive tapenade

Hummus is made from mashed garbanzo beans (also called *chickpeas*). Tapenade is made from pureed olives, capers, and olive oil. These items are usually found in the deli, cheese, or gourmet section of the supermarket.

French toast

1 slice sprouted grain bread

1 egg or ¼ cup Egg Beaters (whites)

1 tablespoon milk (optional)

Dash of cinnamon and/or vanilla extract

2 strawberries

A few drops of olive oil

1. Beat egg in bowl and add milk, cinnamon, and/or vanilla if desired.
2. Soak bread in egg mixture and turn over to saturate both sides of bread as much as possible.
3. Heat pan on stove top and lightly coat with olive oil. Place bread in pan and cook on medium heat, checking the underside for doneness. Flip bread and continue to cook until nice and brown.
4. Remove from heat and layer sliced strawberries on top of the toast. What a way to start the day!

Steel Cut Oats

Makes 4 servings:

¼ cup steel cut oats

½ small apple, chopped

2 tablespoons walnut pieces

Pinch of cinnamon

*Note: Consider making 4 servings at one time (1 cup oats to 4 cups water) to make easy, quick microwave-ready breakfasts.

1. Cook oats in water according to box directions. If preparing more than one serving, refrigerate the excess. Portions can be microwaved later as needed.
2. Apple, walnuts, and cinnamon may be added at the beginning or end of cooking—1/3 cup berries or ½ a pear may be added instead of the ½ apple.

Tune-up Meal Alternates

Grilled Veggie Plate with Meat Garnish and Hummus

1 grilled chicken breast, 3 oz. (or shrimp, or other meat as desired)

½ cup hummus

Roasted mushrooms, broccoli, zucchini, etc. per instructions under roasted vegetables in chapter 21

This is a great way to utilize leftovers from the evening before. Eat your fill of vegetables.

Lentil soup with cabbage slaw

½ cup lentils

Olive oil

2 tomatoes, chopped

1. Sauté lentils in olive oil for 3-4 minutes on medium high heat.
2. Add chopped tomatoes and continue cooking until tomatoes begin to soften.

3. Add 1 cup water and ¼ teaspoon salt. Boil for 20 minutes or until lentils are soft.

Cabbage Slaw

2 cups finely shredded green cabbage
1/2 cup thinly sliced red bell pepper
1/3 cup thinly sliced red onion
2 tablespoons vinaigrette dressing

1. Toss cabbage, bell pepper, onion, vinegar, and oil in a large bowl.
2. Season with salt and pepper; toss again to combine.
3. Enjoy with a bowl of warm lentil soup.

Your own salad creations

See chapter 39 for ideas and let your imagination be your guide.

Fill-up Meal and Side Dish Alternates

Grilled Salmon

1 salmon filet (about the size of your palm). Use wild-caught salmon, if available.
3-4 slices of lemon
3-4 slices of onion
Olive oil
Salt and pepper to taste

1. Heat grill to medium high.
2. Place salmon filet on a piece of aluminum foil skin side down. Drizzle lightly with 1-2 teaspoons of olive oil.

3. Dust salmon with salt and pepper and top with lemon and onion slices.
4. Place the foil in the middle of the grill and close the lid. Let cook for 5 minutes and open lid to check the fish. If it is still raw and opaque-looking, close the lid for another 3-5 minutes.
5. When fish has changed color, check for doneness with a fork—the fish is done when it flakes easily. Be careful not to overcook.
6. Use a knife to peel off the skin while lifting the fish with a spatula. Transfer to a plate and serve.

Note: Try the same recipe under the broiler—place the foil in a baking dish. The general rule for cooking fish, regardless of the cooking method, is 10 minutes of cooking for every inch of thickness. A typical salmon filet takes about 7 minutes.

Fish Taco
3-oz. baked/grilled white fish filet (such as red snapper, trout, halibut, flounder)
Shredded lettuce
Diced tomato
1/4 avocado
1 heaping tablespoon grated cheddar cheese
Juice of half of a lime
Whole grain/low carb tortilla

Place all ingredients in a heated tortilla and squirt with the juice of the lime. Delicious!

Stepped-up Tuna

Note: All tuna has mercury. Canned light tuna is usually skip-jack tuna, which is reported to have less mercury than other tuna species.

2 4 oz. cans chunk light tuna in water, well drained
3 tablespoons olive oil
1 inch ginger root, peeled and chopped into small pieces
1-2 Serrano peppers (or a milder pepper), chopped into small pieces
1 tablespoon chopped garlic (bottled or fresh)
3 tablespoons finely chopped cilantro
1 teaspoon lime juice
Salt
Black pepper

1. Heat the olive oil in a frying pan on medium high. Add ginger, peppers, and garlic and fry for a minute.
2. Reduce heat to medium, add the tuna, and use a flat spatula to stir and break up the tuna meat into small pieces.
3. Add salt and pepper to taste.
4. Cook until tuna is heated through, around 3-4 minutes. Remove from stove top. Immediately add the cilantro and lime juice. Stir vigorously.

This makes many servings, and you can use it more than one way—as the meat part of the fill-up meal, as a filling for half of a toasted sprouted grain pita or tortilla, or as topping for a salad.

Flank Steak with Pesto

Flank steak (4-ounces per serving)

1-2 tablespoons basil pesto (bottled; look in the aisle with spaghetti sauce) or make your own (see recipe below)

Salt and pepper to taste

1. Prepare grill. Place flank steak on grill rack coated with cooking spray and grill 6 minutes on each side or until desired degree of doneness.
2. Cut steak diagonally across grain into thin slices.
3. Drizzle with pesto. Add salt and pepper to taste.

Homemade Pesto

¾ cup fresh cilantro

2 tablespoons slivered almonds, toasted

1 tablespoon chopped, seeded jalapeno pepper

1/8 teaspoon salt

1/8 teaspoon pepper

1 garlic clove, chopped

3 tablespoons plain yogurt

1 ½ teaspoon fresh lime juice

1. Place first 6 ingredients in a blender; process until finely chopped (about 15 seconds).
2. Add yogurt and lime juice; process until smooth.

This makes a great topping for steak, chicken, or fish.

Creamed Spinach

1 10-oz pack of frozen spinach
¼ white onion
¼ cup sour cream
Olive oil
Salt to taste

1. Chop the onion in a food processor, and then fry lightly in two teaspoons of olive oil.
2. Process the spinach in the food processor; add to the onion in the frying pan.
3. Cover and cook at medium-low heat for five minutes (the spinach should not lose its dark green color).
4. Add the sour cream and mix thoroughly. Add salt to taste.

Note: This recipe has sour cream, but it makes more than one serving so the amount of cream per serving is small. Don't cheat!

Kidney Bean Salad

½ teaspoon cumin seeds
1 ½ tablespoons red wine vinegar
1 tablespoon extra-virgin olive oil
1 15-ounce can kidney beans, drained and washed well
¼ cup red onion, finely chopped
1/3 cup walnuts, coarsely chopped
2 tablespoons chopped fresh cilantro

1. Toast the cumin in a skillet over medium heat until fragrant, about 2 minutes.
2. Whisk vinegar and oil in bowl to combine.
3. Combine kidney beans, onion, walnuts, and cilantro in large bowl. Add vinegar and oil mixture. Add the toasted cumin seeds. Toss gently to blend; season with salt and pepper. Makes about 2 servings.

Beans can be used either as the starch or protein part of a fill-up meal or as a topping for a green salad.

Quinoa with a Kick

Note: Natural quinoa has a slightly bitter coating. Unless the quinoa packet states that it is pre-washed, it is prudent to rinse it in water prior to use. Quinoa can be cooked exactly like rice. An electric rice cooker makes it easier to cook quinoa or rice perfectly every time, but using a pot can give just as good results. If all you want is plain quinoa, add one cup of quinoa and two cups of water to a rice cooker and press Cook. However, the recipe below makes quinoa a little more interesting.

1 cup quinoa

1 cup lentils (brown or green)

4 cups water

A handful of grape or cherry tomatoes, or 3 Roma tomatoes chopped into small pieces

1 tablespoon butter

½ cup (or more) meat cut into ½-inch cubes—chicken/sausage/beef/pork (optional).

Salt to taste
Black pepper or ground red pepper to taste
1/2 teaspoonful *garam masala* (optional)
Note: *garam masala* is a spice mix from India available in all Indian grocery stores and sometimes in the Asian section of supermarkets. It is extremely high in antioxidants.

1. Rinse the quinoa in a rice cooker and drain well. Add the lentils and mix.
2. Add the water, tomatoes, meat, butter, salt, and pepper. Start the rice cooker. When the quinoa is almost done, add the *garam masala*, if desired.

Enjoy. Remember to fill only one-third of your plate.

Baked Sprouted Grain Chips
1 sprouted grain tortilla

1. Place tortilla on a paper plate in the microwave and cook on full power for 45 seconds on each side or until crisp. Note: Microwave ovens vary widely in power, so keep a close eye on the tortilla to make sure it does not burn. You may also need more than 45 seconds on each side to crisp the tortilla.
2. OR Pre-heat a conventional oven to 325 degrees F. Place the tortilla directly on the middle rack of the oven. Bake 5 minutes. Flip tortilla over and continue to bake an

additional 2 minutes. Watch carefully. As soon as the tortilla begins to brown, remove from oven to cool.

3. Break into chip-size pieces. Enjoy half a tortilla with salsa, hummus, or guacamole as a mid-morning or pre-dinner snack.

Tasty Sprouted Mung Beans

Whole mung beans can be obtained from any Indian grocery store or from the Asian section of many supermarkets.

1 cup sprouted mung beans (see sprouting instructions below)
1 teaspoon finely chopped or grated garlic
1 teaspoon finely chopped or grated ginger
A few sprigs of cilantro, coarsely chopped
1 teaspoon cumin seeds
1 tablespoon canola or other oil
Salt to taste

1. Heat the oil in a frying pan until it is very hot.
2. Add the ginger and garlic and fry lightly.
3. Add 1 teaspoon cumin seeds.
4. When the cumin seeds turn brown, add the sprouted beans.
5. Add salt. Turn off heat, stir, and garnish with cilantro leaves.

Use the beans as a snack or as the starch or protein part of a fill-up meal.

Sprouting Mung Beans:

1. Spread half a bowl of dry mung beans on a plate. Pick through and remove any stones.
2. Put back in the bowl, rinse, and discard the rinse water.
3. Add fresh water to cover the beans by an inch.
4. Cover the bowl and soak the beans overnight on the kitchen counter.
5. Next morning, drain the water.
6. Replace the cover and leave on the counter for 24-36 hours. The beans will have sprouted by then. Note: you are not looking for long sprouts, ¼-inch is sufficient.
7. Place in the refrigerator until ready to cook.

Plain sprouted mung beans can be used as a snack or added to scrambled eggs to provide texture.

Part 5:

Hanging Tough— The Next Six Months

You have made it through the first two weeks.

You have lost weight. You feel better and have more energy. Your sleep more soundly and wake up rested.

You have a tasty low-glycemic breakfast every morning, mid-morning and pre-dinner snacks, and a tune-up meal and a fill-up meal daily. You eat slowly, letting your hunger guide your food intake.

You have learned to prepare your meals without excess salt, spices, or sugar, using mostly natural, unprocessed foods and just enough fat or oil to make the food appealing without being unhealthy.

Your addictive cravings have disappeared, though you still have occasional empty-stomach hunger. Your palate now appreciates the taste and texture of natural foods—the sweetness of a ripe tomato, the crispy crunch of lettuce, the tangy bite of a radish.

You have taken huge steps towards a healthier lifestyle, but challenges lie ahead. The first of these is the responsibility you face today. For the past two weeks, you were able to follow the step-by-step menus and recipes in the book. Now you have to use your new knowledge and experience to develop your own menus and recipes. But not to worry; as you will see in the next chapter, the transition does not have to be abrupt.

You will face other challenges. You will have to navigate your way through a world filled with tempting foods and stay "on program" at parties and weddings and at Christmas and Thanksgiving and other celebrations. You will have to plan your eating carefully on out-of-town trips. When life becomes stressful, you will have to curb your desire for comfort foods. You will have to be patient during plateaus—those frustrating days and weeks in which you don't lose weight in spite of doing all the right things.

This section will help you anticipate and overcome ten common obstacles you are likely to face. You should come back to these pages over and over again. The challenges and solutions in this section are distilled from the real-life experience of hundreds of people. The more times you read these tips, the more they will become a part of you and the more you will appreciate them. Also, many of the weight-loss secrets that you read about in Part II of this book are put into practice here.

Chapter 23

Challenge #1—Maintaining Your Momentum

The well-ordered eating plan you followed in the first two weeks has ended. You are on now on your own. If you enjoy cooking, you are probably looking forward to developing your own recipes and exploring new tastes.

But if you don't like to cook, you run the risk of getting stuck in a rut, of repeating the recipes from the first two weeks over and over again. You will get bored, and being bored with your food is the first step towards straying from the program.

The good news is this transition need not be scary. Here's what you should do.

Eating schedule

1. Plan, plan, plan. You must spend a few minutes every day putting together the menu for the next day. It is impossible to stress this enough. The day you stop planning is the day you set yourself up for failure. Remember—the food world out there is designed to tempt you, to catch you in an unguarded moment

and trip you up. Like an explorer entering unknown territory, you have to take every step with forethought and deliberation.

By the evening of each day, you should know what you are going to have for every meal and snack the next day. All food items should be on hand, all food preparation completed. If you are going to eat out, visualize yourself sitting at a restaurant and ordering your meal. Decide which food items will you select, and what will you absolutely stay away from. The more concrete your plan for the next day, the more likely you are to stick to it.

2. Make sure you continue to have breakfast, the mid-morning snack, a tune-up meal, the pre-dinner snack, and a fill-up meal daily. Do not skip a meal or snack even if you have no hunger. Skipping one of these will just make you more hungry later in the day, or even the next day, and you will find it harder to stick to the program. Another reason to eat all your meals is to keep reassuring your body there is plenty of food available so it will be less reluctant to give up its stored fat. Remember—hunger is the enemy of weight loss.

Menus and recipes

1. Keep using the recipes from the first two weeks, including those from the alternate recipes section. In fact, you can continue to use the breakfast and snack items from the first two weeks for as long as you want. But you should start adding new lunch and dinner recipes so you don't get bored. A couple of new recipes a week is a good start. By the end of four to six weeks, at least half your lunches and dinners should be your

own recipes. This variety will keep you looking forward to your next meal with enthusiasm.

2. There are three sections in this book that will help you with new recipes. Start by checking out chapter 37, "Food Choices after the First Two Weeks." This section explores every food group—vegetables, meat, dairy, etc. Use food items from this list as inspirations for your own recipes.

Note: Make sure to read about fruits in chapter 37. Fruits are an important part of a healthy eating plan, but you have to make the right choices. Some fruits have more goodness and fewer calories than others. In chapter 37 you will learn about juicy fruits and crunchy fruits, citrus fruits and berries. You will also find suggestions for desserts, and how to sensibly use alcohol while trying to lose weight.

In chapter 38 you will find ten each of dinner (fill-up meal) and lunch (tune-up meal) recipes. The recipes are designed so leftovers from dinner become part of the next day's lunch.

Chapter 39 is the "Salad" section. This chapter offers suggestions for putting together simple but tasty salads. Fruits, berries, mushrooms, cucumber, radishes, and of course, beans, cheese, and meats allow for infinite variety. Salads are great tune-up meals. You will also find that you lose weight faster when one of your daily meals is a salad.

Eating pace

1. Remember to eat slowly. Take about twenty minutes to finish lunch and dinner, especially if a second helping is available. If you cannot eat slowly, that's OK; just don't take a second helping

until twenty minutes have gone by. If you are still hungry after twenty minutes, go ahead and have that second helping, but...

2. Make sure you are taking the second helping to satisfy hunger, not to indulge desire. This is a real risk if you make your food too tasty. Save the spices and special touches for free-styling days. On other days, keep your food natural and simple.

Doctor Alok says:

- Plan, plan, plan.
- Continue to eat five times a day, hungry or not.
- Introduce new menu items.
- Remember to eat slowly.

Chapter 24

Challenge #2—Cheating Sensibly

A sensible eating regimen is more sustainable if it allows for a treat now and then. After the first two weeks are over you can occasionally eat something you really enjoy but would ordinarily be off-limits on the program. I call this "freestyling," a concept you first read about in chapter 15. Having some flexibility in your eating choices makes it easier to stay on the program.

There are rules for freestyling—you don't want to overdo it, and you especially don't want to risk re-addiction. It is okay to go to the zoo, but make sure there are bars between you and the tiger!

The rules:

1. A freestyling meal is a modified fill-up meal. The meal should have the usual meat and vegetables (with each conforming to a third-of-a-plate serving size), but it can have two additional items. One of the two items replaces the low-glycemic starch on the plate with any food or drink of your choice, and the other is a freebie, which can also be anything. Each of these should be a reasonable serving-size portion. Within these guidelines you have a lot of flexibility in your choice of the two items. You can

enjoy half a baked potato (item 1) and a piece of cake (item 2) to go along with your steak and vegetables, or have apple pie (item 1) with ice cream (item 2).

You can get creative—a small hamburger, medium fries, and a salad is a perfectly acceptable freestyling meal. The hamburger patty is the meat, the salad is the vegetable, the hamburger bun is item 1, and the fries are item 2. A couple of slices of pizza or two glasses of wine are also acceptable freestyling items. Use your imagination, but make sure you have your meat (or other protein, such as beans or a soy preparation) and your veggies along with the freestyling items. To repeat, a freestyling meal cannot consist *only* of the forbidden items. Wolfing down a half-gallon of ice cream or a large bag of potato chips is not a freestyling meal.

2. You can have two freestyling meals a week, with two to three days between each of the two meals. Wednesday and Saturday or Thursday and Sunday are good choices because you can have a freestyling meal over the weekend. But you can use any two-day pair with the required gaps between the days.

You should stick to the same days from week to week; you can't declare a day to be a freestyling day just because you find yourself in a restaurant. Of course, it is quite acceptable to occasionally juggle a freestyling day because of a special event such as a wedding or anniversary. But don't move your freestyling days around casually or you might find yourself freestyling three or four times a week. Note: After the first six to eight weeks, many people are comfortable freestyling just once a week. By this time you will be able to judge what works best for you.

3. There are two reasons for the two-or-three-day gap between freestyling meals. First, freestyling on successive days can rekindle addictive hunger. Second, if you have been eating correctly on the days before a freestyling meal, you will have room in your glycogen tank to catch some extra glucose calories without having them spill over into the fat tank. But if you freestyle two days in a row, you will fill your glycogen tank on the first day and spill calories into the fat tank on the second day.

4. It is best to have the freestyling meal at a restaurant so you don't bring tempting foods into your house. If you do want to eat at home, you should have just enough freestyling food available for one meal. You cannot buy a whole pie, eat a slice, and keep the rest in the refrigerator for the next freestyling day. You cannot buy a tub of ice-cream thinking you will have a couple of scoops today and save the rest for later. You know exactly what is going to happen—you will eat the leftover pie or ice-cream when you should not. Don't expose yourself to temptation.

5. You should not use trigger foods as part of a freestyling meal. Trigger foods are foods that make you lose control. Most of us have a trigger food or two; you know what yours are. It may be ice cream or potato chips or salted nuts or chocolate candy, to name a few. If you absolutely want to risk a small portion of a trigger food, eat it at the end of a meal and make sure a second helping is not available.

6. A weight gain of one to two pounds is to be expected after a freestyling meal. This is not fat. Most of this weight is either retained water (if there was extra salt in the meal) and/or glycogen. For every ounce of glucose that is stored as

glycogen, the body has to retain three to four ounces of water, so the glycogen weight adds up quickly. You should lose all of this weight, and a little more, before the next freestyling day comes around. If you don't, then skip the next freestyling meal and cut back on the subsequent freestyling portions.

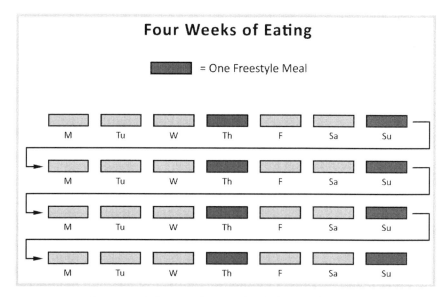

Figure 11. A typical freestyling schedule. Only one freestyling meal is allowed on a freestyling day—either lunch or dinner.

Doctor Alok says:

- A freestyling meal is a fill-up meal in which the low-glycemic carb is replaced with a food of your choice, and there is an additional freebie. These two items can be any food or drink, but the portion size should be reasonable.
- Have a freestyling meal twice a week, on the same two days of every week.

- Keep a two-to-three-day gap between freestyling meals.
- Stay away from your trigger foods.
- Don't keep leftover freestyling foods at home—you will eat them at the wrong time.
- You should lose the weight you gain after a freestyling meal, and a little more, before the next freestyling meal comes around.

Chapter 25

Challenge #3—Counting Every Success

This program has two goals. The first is to eat correctly; the second is to lose weight. Each of the two goals will improve your health independent of the other, *so success in either is a success.* Think about this: eating better is not just a tool for weight loss; eating better is an important goal in its own right.

There is an important difference between the two goals. Eating better is under your control. How much weight you lose as a result of eating correctly is *not* under your control. As you know by now, weight loss is not just about calories in and calories out, or eating less and exercising more. Your body also has a say in the matter because it can slow down its metabolism, conserve its calories, and fight the weight loss. You have no control over this.

It makes absolutely no sense to judge your success or failure by the rate of weight loss, but that's what everyone does. When the weight loss temporarily stops in spite of doing all the right things (a common occurrence), the tendency is to become frustrated and fall off the wagon.

But there is a second approach—you can stay focused on eating correctly and accept any weight loss as only a side-benefit. Once your cravings are gone you have control over what you eat. If you continue to eat correctly, you will lose weight; you just cannot control how much and how fast. It is unrealistic to insist your body lose weight at a rate that keeps you happy. The reality is that your body will lose weight at a rate that keeps *it* happy.

So, the right question to ask every morning is, "Did I eat correctly yesterday—and do I have a plan for eating correctly today"? If the answer to both questions is yes, then you have won yesterday's battle and you will win today's battle. Do this every day and you will stay on the road to better health. "Did my body lose any weight today?" is a secondary question. If it did, fine; if not, it means your body is doing its own thing. Let it be. Do not measure your success by a result over which you have no control. Become fixated on the weight loss and you risk becoming frustrated and squandering all the gains you have worked so hard for. Be patient, and your body will come around.

Of course, it is only natural to want to track your weight. This brings up another question: How often should you weigh yourself? There is no hard and fast rule. For at least the first few weeks, it is useful to check your weight every morning. Each of us is different, and keeping a close eye on your weight (be consistent as to the time you weigh) will help you learn how your body responds to different foods. So weigh yourself daily and keep a record. It is best to keep your weight diary next to the scale so you can enter the date and the weight immediately after weighing. You do not even have to use a diary; a 3" X 5" card and a pencil will do the job. Just make sure you keep the cards together in a safe place as they fill up.

It is very important to weigh yourself if you have eaten anything off-program the previous day. Write down your exact "sin" right next to your weight; it is a valuable learning experience. Daily weighing also helps you fine-tune your freestyling. Put an asterisk next to your weight on the day immediately following each freestyling meal. And, as I said in the previous chapter, if you have not lost the weight gained after a freestyling meal before the next freestyling meal comes around, you need to skip the next freestyling meal—and eat less food or different foods when you freestyle again.

Expect the weight loss to slow down after the first couple of weeks. There is no right amount of weight to lose every week— everyone is different—but you should lose some weight every week, even if it is just half a pound. If you are not losing any weight at all, then you have hit a plateau—see chapter 26.

Doctor Alok says:

- Eating correctly is under your control; how much weight you lose is not.
- Judge your success by whether or not you are eating correctly. If you judge your success by how much weight you are losing, you are setting yourself up for disappointment.
- Keep a record of your weight, your transgressions, and your freestyling days.

Chapter 26

Challenge #4—Being Patient During Plateaus

No one really knows why a person who is steadily losing weight suddenly stops doing so, but this a common experience. Is it because the person has become lax about sticking to the eating program? Is it because of a slowing down of the metabolism? Or is it a combination of the two?

The first thing to do when you hit a plateau is to take an honest look at how well you are staying on the program. Are you beginning to cut corners? Has that glass of wine on a free-styling day turned into a glass of wine every day? Are you snacking on foods you should not be snacking on? Are you eating too much of the program foods, so that twenty almonds have now become forty? Or are you not eating enough, skipping the morning or the pre-dinner snack—or even worse, are you skipping meals? This is an easy trap to fall into because you will not have much hunger. However, not eating enough, or not eating *often* enough may force the body to slow down the metabolism—and you don't want that.

So, if you are not eating correctly, go back and re-adjust your eating program.

But if you *are* eating correctly, then the body is responsible for the plateau. A simplistic way to look at plateaus is to compare a lifetime's accumulation of fat to the growth rings in a tree trunk. Some rings are wider than others, depending on how much the tree was able to grow that year, and the innermost rings are the oldest. In the same way, most of us do not put on fat at a steady rate. There might be an uptick in weight gain during college days, another right after getting married, perhaps another during a period of work or family stress. Think of each recent layer of fat as being "softer" than the deeper, older layer next to it. The older the layer of fat, the "harder" it is.

As weight loss starts, imagine the body going through the most recent and softest fat first, then hesitating for a while before it breaks through into the next, harder, layer and then the next. Each plateau represents this hesitation.

It is also possible that the older the fat, the less blood supply it has—after all, it has been sitting around doing nothing—and it takes longer for the body to start moving it out of storage and using it up. Either way, weight loss slows down for a while before it picks up again. When you do break through a plateau, don't be surprised if you lose two or three pounds in just a couple of days. We see this often in our weight management program but don't know why it happens. The point is, just as weight gain usually occurs in fits and starts, so does weight loss.

The first plateau may occur at a month or two. Stay on the program, and you will start losing weight again in a few days or a week. Subsequent plateaus are longer until a permanent plateau is reached. If you reach a plateau you just cannot break through, it means your body is not ready to lose any more weight at this time. Recent research shows that, as weight loss continues, the body begins to slow down its metabolism. The body assumes there is a famine and is trying to help you live longer by using fewer calories. But, for a person trying to lose weight, this can be extremely frustrating because the weight loss comes to a halt. If you try to push harder, you will just get hungry and this may make the body hunker down even more. Accept this plateau weight; you have reached a new balance between your eating and your metabolism. In fact, if you have stopped losing weight in spite of doing all the right things and are constantly hungry, it is probably a good idea to let your body regain 3-4 percent of your starting weight—see the box in chapter 33. The good news is you are likely to reach the weight loss goal you set in Part III before you reach a permanent plateau.

Will you ever break through this plateau? Probably so, but there is not enough research to say how long this might take. People are different. Focus on eating correctly, celebrate the weight you have lost, and you will find your own answer.

Doctor Alok says:

- Plateaus are a normal part of the weight-loss journey.
- If you hit a plateau, make sure you are eating correctly.
- If you are eating correctly, be patient and you will break through the plateau.
- If, in spite of doing everything right, you just cannot break through a plateau, accept your new, lower weight. You have reached a new balance between your eating and your metabolism.

Chapter 27

Challenge #5—The Late-Night Refrigerator Raid

Do you often find yourself sneaking into the kitchen late at night looking for something to eat?

Eating late at night can undo all your hard work from the rest of the day. Late night cravings are usually for foods that will hit the spot. Chips, nuts, ice cream, a cold slice of pizza, even cereal with milk and sugar—not only are these foods packed with calories, they can also re-kindle your addiction.

First, you should go through your refrigerator and pantry one more time and make sure there is nothing there that calls out to you. You did this once already when you started the program, but forbidden foods tend to creep in. Make sure other family members are not sabotaging you!

Next, pre-cut a few pieces of a hard cheese—cheddar works great—and leave them in your refrigerator. Each piece should be about an ounce. In the USA, hard cheddar is available as a 1" X 2" X 6" block. A ½-inch slice of this is about an ounce. When you have a late-night snack attack, go into the kitchen, extract one (and only one) piece of cheese from the refrigerator, take it back to bed, and nibble on it slowly. Hard cheese has a great mouthfeel and enough salt, fat, and protein to hit whatever spot you are trying to hit. Your cravings will be gone in a few minutes. Now go to sleep.

Two notes of caution: First, make sure you cut the cheese slices ahead of time. If you cut a slice during a snack attack, it is likely to be a two-inch rather than a half-inch slice. Second, take the cheese back to the bedroom to eat. If you eat it in the kitchen, you will be tempted to grab a second piece.

My Son and I

When I first put myself on this program, I took my own advice and cleared out my fridge and pantry. Of course, that did not break my late-night snacking habit. Every so often I would wander into the kitchen late at night looking for something to eat, and I would find one of my teenage sons on the same quest. We would do a thorough search, hoping against hope that I had missed something during my housecleaning rounds. Of course, I had not. We would finally give up, smile rue-fully at each other, and go back to bed.

Doctor Alok says:

- If you are prone to raiding the refrigerator at night, a small piece of cheese is a great late-night snack.

Chapter 28

Challenge #6—When the Tiger Pounces

You are at the office. A co-worker comes by. "It's Kathy's birthday today," she says, "We have a cake for her. Come and sing 'Happy Birthday.'" You walk over to the break room. A luscious triple layer chocolate cake is unveiled. A colleague passes you a slice. You accept it mindlessly and pick up a fork…

STOP! You are facing the tiger. Use the mantra you learned in chapter 11. Look at the cake and repeat the following words slowly to yourself five times: "This is the tiger—*but I am stronger.*"

When confronted by an attractive but forbidden food, the desire-driven impulsive mind can push aside the rational mind and make you lose control. However, the few seconds it takes for you to repeat your mantra five times will be enough to snap you back into reality and give you the strength to resist.

Think about the difference between pleasure and happiness. If you eat that slice of cake, you will have a few minutes of pleasure—but you will not be happy because you know you did the wrong thing. However, if you decide not to eat the cake, you will give up a few minutes of pleasure but gain hours of happiness because you have won yet another battle.

It's your choice.

Doctor Alok says:

- Beware of the tiger! It will ambush you when you are least expecting it. Repeat the mantra five times and beat back the tiger.
- There is a difference between pleasure and happiness. Succumbing to the tiger might give you a few minutes of pleasure (followed by guilt); fighting off the tiger will give you long-lasting happiness.

Chapter 29

Challenge #7—Business Travel

Business travel is not a vacation. It is a part of your professional life and should not be used as an excuse to go off-program.

That said, business travel *is* a high-risk time for not eating correctly. You are tired after being cooped up in a car or airplane for hours. You are in an unfamiliar town on an empty stomach. You are out of your daily routine. And you may be anticipating a stressful meeting the next day. It is easy to falter.

Don't do it. You will regret it later.

The key to eating correctly on a business trip is to make a detailed eating plan ahead of time and stick to it.

Before you leave:

1. Write down every meal you anticipate eating. If your trip is longer than three days, write down the meals for at least the first three days. You can plan out the remaining days later.

2. Think about the circumstance and content of every meal. Where will you have breakfast, lunch, and dinner? If you are going to be on your own for any of these meals, get on the Internet and make a list of sensible eating places close to your hotel (see also "Challenge #9—Eating Out" in chapter 31). For

example, as I write these words I know I will be staying overnight at a hotel in downtown Chicago next week. I did a search
for nearby Mediterranean restaurants and found four within
easy walking distance of where I'm staying. I have looked at the
reviews and I already know which one I am going to eat at.

3. If you are going to be eating out with business associ-
ates, visualize ahead of time what kind of food you are going
to order and even more important, what you will definitely stay
away from. This includes avoiding white bread and other white
flour products such as tortillas and chips; potatoes, white rice,
and, of course, dessert if it is a non-freestyling day.

4. Make up mini-packs of twenty almonds or ten walnut
halves to take with you. Keep a couple of packs handy at all
times. Use this food liberally, along with fruit or cheese (if
available). You can double up on your snacks, if necessary. Also
make sure you eat something from your snack-pack a half-hour
before lunch and dinner.

5. For the first day, prepare two sprouted grain or whole
wheat sandwiches before you leave. Eat the sandwiches during
your travel on the first day. If possible, eat at least one sandwich
thirty minutes to an hour before you arrive at your destination.
By doing this, you will not find yourself in an unfamiliar town
on an empty stomach—a dangerous combination. If you are
driving, you may want to go a step further and take an insu-
lated cooler with bread, sandwich materials, salad, and even a
pre-prepared meal or two.

6. Call ahead and find hotels that provide a refrigerator in
the room. Many hotels now offer this amenity. Even if this not
standard for the hotel, most will place a refrigerator (and even

a microwave) in the room upon prior request. If you brought food with you, transfer it to the refrigerator. If not, go shopping and get some fruit and cheese to put in the refrigerator.

7. Now go have supper—you already know where you are going to eat, right?

Get a good night's sleep. You are all set to stay in control.

Doctor Alok says:

- Business travel is not an excuse to go off-program.
- The secret to success is the same on a business trip as it is for the program—plan every meal ahead of time.

Chapter 30

Challenge #8—Vacations

If you want to stay on program during your vacation, use the business travel section (chapter 29) to plan your eating. But vacations are meant to be enjoyed, and it is OK to loosen up a little. Even so, it is best do some planning so you do not totally decompensate.

1. Just as with business travel, make up mini-packs of twenty almonds or ten walnut halves. Keep a couple of packs handy at all times. Use these for snacking, along with fruit and cheese (instead of pastries and chips). Make sure you have a snack thirty minutes before lunch and dinner.

2. Plan to have one major meal a day that fits the program guidelines, preferably a tune-up meal; you will feel better for it. The other meal can be your "vacation experience" meal. Enjoy the local cuisine, but in moderation.

3. Stay active. Walk, walk, then walk some more.

4. When you get back home, do at least three days of the "first two weeks" program in chapters 19 and 20. This will get you de-addicted and back on the wagon. If you can do a whole week, you will also get rid of any weight you put on. Stick to the program without cutting corners—it is better to do three

days correctly than to do a week during which you are cheating every day. Have your program breakfast, lunch, dinner, and the two snacks. Don't skip meals or try to go on a diet. You will likely find it hard to control your hunger and it might take longer to turn things around.

Doctor Alok says:

- A little loosening up on vacation is OK, but do not go completely off-program.
- Use snack-packs liberally between meals.
- A minimum of one meal daily should be a program meal.
- As soon as you are back home, do at least three days of the "first two weeks" program to de-addict and get back on track.

Chapter 31

Challenge #9—Eating Out

When eating out, the most dangerous foods are white starch (with or without fat) and sugar. Examples include bread, tortillas (flour and corn), bagels, chips, pita bread, white rice, pizza, pasta (except in limited amounts—a third of a plate), and, of course, dessert—cakes, pies, and ice cream.

If possible, eat a little something before leaving for the restaurant. Twenty almonds or ten walnut halves with a small piece of cheese, or half an apple or a few strawberries works well. This will take the edge off your appetite and lessen the temptation to make bad food choices. Use the same tactic before a party.

If possible, decide on what you are going to order *before* you enter the restaurant.

Some Suggestions When Eating Out

Mediterranean/Middle Eastern/Greek: Send back the pita bread. Start with a cup of lentil soup. For the main course, a nice Greek salad with feta cheese and grilled chicken or lamb is perfect. A couple of falafel (garbanzo bean patties) is a nice accompaniment.

Italian: Send back the rolls. Start with a salad and a cup of minestrone soup. Take your time over these so the edge is off your hunger. For the main course, choose something with meat and with a limited amount of white flour. If you are having pasta, remember the one-third of a plate rule. Put the extra pasta in a take-out box, or even better, send it back so you do not have access to it. Go crazy on the marinara sauce—it has anti-oxidants and is good for you. Some restaurants will put grilled salmon on the pasta; otherwise topping it with a couple of meatballs is fine. Stay away from the pizza, calzones, and Italian subs.

Mexican: Don't eat the chips! Also, send back the tortillas. Have the fajita plate; it usually comes with some veggies mixed in with the meat. Ask for extra veggies with the fajitas. Have the rice as long as you also have whole beans (not refried beans). Adding the beans to the rice lowers the glycemic index of the rice because of the soluble fiber in the beans (see chapter 9 for more on soluble fiber).

Chinese: If you are not on a salt-restricted diet, start with a cup of wonton or egg drop soup; if you need to restrict salt, you should not be in a Chinese restaurant in the first place. You may also be able to find an entrée-size soup on the menu that has lots of veggies, meat, and shrimp. Otherwise, steamed food is best; moo-goo gai pan is also good. Your next choice is any other stir-fried food without sauce. Ask the server to substitute a cup of noodles for the rice because noodles have a lower glycemic index than the short-grain rice served in Chinese restaurants. Stay away from batter-fried or heavily sauced foods.

American/Steakhouse: Send back the bread. Have a small steak with a double order of vegetables. As an accompaniment, have mushrooms or a small serving of rice instead of a baked potato/mashed potatoes/potatoes au gratin. If you must have the baked potato, eat only half.

Doctor Alok says:

- Eat something before going out to eat.
- Know what you are going to order before you enter the restaurant.
- Send back anything made from processed starch, and skip the dessert.

Chapter 32

Challenge #10—Alcohol

The good news is that alcohol cannot be turned into fat. The bad news is that alcohol frees up other foods to be turned into fat.

The body appears to use alcohol in preference to other fuels as an energy source. This means that if alcohol is available, the two more commonly used fuels—glucose and fat—are shunted directly into storage. Every alcohol calorie potentially frees up a glucose or fat calorie to go into the fat tank.

A jigger (1 ½ ounces) of 80 proof liquor such as whisky or gin contains about one hundred calories. A can of beer or a five-ounce serving of wine has approximately one hundred and fifty calories. A couple of drinks a day—beer, wine, or hard liquor—can add up in a hurry.

While some studies suggest a slight reduction in heart disease from moderate alcohol consumption (one drink a day for women and one to two drinks a day for men), the American Heart Association does not recommend the use of alcohol for this purpose. Other studies also suggest a health benefit specifically from drinking red wine, but the evidence is not strong.

It is possible that red wine drinkers have other lifestyle habits that promote good health.

The bottom line: Drinking a little bit of alcohol may be good for the heart, but losing weight is even better. If you use alcohol at all, use it as part of a freestyling meal (see chapter 24). If you must have alcohol on other days, confine yourself to no more than one glass of wine or one drink. But if you find you are having trouble losing weight—cut out the alcohol. You will not be sorry.

Doctor Alok says:

- Alcohol contains empty calories.
- Use alcohol only as part of a freestyling meal.

Part 6:

Taking Control of The Rest of Your Life

Take a moment to celebrate your achievements over the past six months.

You have lost weight. You have become an educated consumer of food. Your taste spectrum has expanded so you enjoy simple meals made from wholesome, natural ingredients. You have newfound confidence in your ability to make the right eating choices. Your health has improved. You have more energy. You feel good about yourself.

The challenge now is to hold on to your gains. It is easy to gradually lose focus, to become lax in sticking to the program. If this happens, the weight will start to come back. You have invested many months in getting to where you are today; you cannot afford to backslide. Eating healthy, keeping off the weight you have lost, and taking responsibility for your health has to become a way of life for the rest of your life. It will help if you:

a) Have a clear sense of purpose (what am I doing and why am I doing it?);

b) Partner with your physician to take ownership of some important "health numbers"; and

c) Reduce the amount of stress in your life, because stress is the enemy of healthy eating.

I'll expand on each of these ideas in the next few chapters.

Chapter 33

Living With a Clear
Sense of Purpose

Two roads diverged in a wood, and I—
I took the one less traveled by,
And that has made all the difference.

Robert Frost, 1920

For the person who is committed to eating differently and maintaining a healthy weight, these words say it all. While so many other people are walking down one road, you have chosen to walk the other—the road less traveled, the road of health—and this will make a difference to the rest of your life.

Think about this. Until a few thousand years ago, there really was a "road" most of humanity walked along. This road meandered through the forests and grasslands from which came our food—fruits and roots and leaves and meat. Not only did we gather our food directly from nature, we were also a part of nature. Our food and our bodies fit each together like matched pieces of a jigsaw puzzle.

But then we began to separate ourselves from nature. We no longer lived *in* nature, we lived *on* nature. We began to manipulate nature to our wishes. As an early step in this changing relationship, we started to control our food. Instead of accepting what was naturally available, we learned to grow what we desired. Grain became an increasingly important part of our diet. We also began to raise goats and sheep and cattle for milk and meat. We became the only mammal to drink milk after being weaned, and the only mammal to drink the milk of another species. We began to veer off the road we had walked on for so long.

As the next step, we learned how to make our food taste better. Cooking oil, butter, sugar, salt, and spices are all recent entries into the kitchen. We do not need any of these five to stay in good health. This applies even to salt; the human body needs much less salt than the teaspoonful or two most of us are used to eating every day (see chapter 36 for more on salt). The main purpose of the five additions to our cooking repertoire is to make food tastier and to encourage us to eat beyond hunger—to eat for pleasure, for the satisfaction of desire.

Now we are at the third step in the great changing of our food. Today's technology allows us to turn natural food into unnatural food products. The body has no prior experience in handling these highly altered products and often cannot handle them without getting hurt. Some of the alteration begins very early in the life of the food. For example, we get our meat and milk from cattle that are fed corn instead of grass; this increases the amount of saturated fat in the meat and unfavorably affects the ratio of omega-3 to omega-6 fatty acids. Some of the alteration occurs after the food is gathered—we grind grain into a fine powder and discard the bran, raising the glycemic index and eliminating all fiber. And some of the things we eat have no connection to nature at all—artificial sweeteners, dyes, preservatives…the list goes on.

We have now left the road our ancestors walked for thousands of generations. Instead, we find ourselves on a new road that is lined not with trees but with bright neon signs that draw us towards highly altered but extremely tasty designer foods. This road meanders not through forests and grasslands but through feedlots and factories that pour out vast quantities of altered foods that are great for profit, but not for health.

You are among the few who have decided to ignore the neon signs that line this new road. You looked ahead to where the road was leading, and you did not like what you saw—obesity, hypertension, diabetes, heart disease, stroke, and cancer. So you made a choice. You turned around and walked back to that original road, the road of our ancestors, the one we should never have left. You, along with a few others, are now walking this road less traveled; the road that leads us back to nature and away from the ills caused by today's foods. This is the road you will walk for the rest of your life.

Most of your food shopping is done in the fruit and vegetable section of the supermarket, with perhaps a brief stop at the butcher's counter to pick up some lean meat or fish. You know when and where the local farmers' markets are held, and you go there as often as you can to get fresh, locally grown produce.

You start the day with a simple, low-glycemic breakfast. One of your major daily meals is heavy on colorful veggies and fruits—either a salad, or lightly cooked vegetables—along with beans, cheese, and perhaps a little meat. The other is a plated meal of modest proportions with protein such as meat, beans, or tofu; a generous serving of vegetables; and a moderate portion of caged carbohydrate. You eat this meal slowly, letting your hunger be your guide. If twenty minutes after you started eating you are still hungry, you take a second helping.

You keep small snacks handy and use them to cut down your hunger between lunch and dinner. Every few days you eat something extra-special, avoiding, of course, your trigger foods. You are either slowly losing weight or have reached a stable plateau.

Once in a while you still have to fight the tiger of temptation, and sometimes it sneaks through your defenses. But you soon shoo it out. If you don't, you immediately begin to sense the physical changes from eating the wrong foods, especially the swings in your blood sugar level that leave you tired and listless. Your body has become used to wholesome food and it can tell the difference. You need to quickly get back on track.

Of course, the tiger never goes away for good. A prolonged life-stress, a vacation, or a long business trip with too many restaurant meals can bring back the cravings of addiction. The good news is you know how to de-addict. A few days or a week of the "First two weeks" program and you are back in control.

Your new lifestyle will have far-reaching effects. Ten, twenty, thirty years later your health is likely to be better, your enjoyment of life greater. So that is your purpose—to make every remaining day of your life a healthier, happier one.

Have you regained some of your lost weight?

If you have lost 10 percent or more of your starting weight, it is not unusual to regain a few pounds before you settle down at a steady weight. Your body and you are negotiating a weight at which both are happy. This is actually a good thing; recent research suggests that going down to the lowest possible weight and trying to stay there encourages your body to fight back by drastically slowing your metabolism and increasing your hunger. So, making peace with your body is a good thing.

That said, the weight regain should not be more than about 3-4 percent of the original weight—if a 200-pound person loses 30 pounds (a 15 percent weight loss), the weight regain should not be more than 6-8 pounds.

Doctor Alok says:

- You have invested so much time and effort in getting to where you are—don't start backsliding.
- You are walking the road less traveled—the road that leads to health.
- The tiger never leaves. Beware of temptation.

Chapter 34

Partnering With Your Physician and Owning Your Health Numbers

Having a clear sense of purpose focuses the mind, but you also have to look after your body. Losing weight is likely to add years to your life. You need to make these extra years as healthy as possible. Your goal is to extend your *healthspan* along with your lifespan.

You have to anticipate and avoid potential health problems. There are five numbers that can help you monitor your body and warn you of problems down the road. Two of these are your weight and blood pressure, and the other three are blood tests. Each of these is an indicator of a condition known as the metabolic syndrome. Having the metabolic syndrome greatly increases the risk of health problems in the future, so you need to know the answer to each of these questions:

- Is your BMI more than thirty?
- Do you have high blood pressure?

The next three are blood tests:
- Your fasting blood glucose (blood sugar) level. Is it too high?
- Your triglyceride level. Is it too high?
- Your high-density lipoprotein (HDL) cholesterol level (the good cholesterol). Is it too low?

A yes to any three of the questions is enough to make a diagnosis of metabolic syndrome. Of course, even if one of these numbers is abnormal there is cause for concern, but a combination of three or more raises a *huge* red flag. For some people, it may not be possible to bring the BMI below thirty even after losing weight—and that's OK, as long as the lost weight is not coming back. But that still leaves four other numbers to try and bring into the normal range.

Understanding and taking ownership of these numbers will help you get the full benefit of weight loss by allowing you to monitor the health of your body. Even if all the numbers (other than your weight) were normal before you started the program, it is still important to keep an eye on them because they can start moving into the red zone as the years go by.

If some of the numbers were not normal before you lost weight, they are likely to have improved. But weight loss alone may not bring the numbers completely back to normal, especially in those of us who are older or if the numbers were very abnormal to begin with. Also, some of us have a genetic tendency to high blood pressure, diabetes, or bad cholesterol numbers. Weight loss certainly helps, but it may also be necessary for your doctor to prescribe medications to bring the numbers into the normal range.

Let's look at each of the five numbers:

Weight: You are already an expert on this. To re-state an important point: it is not necessary to be at some ideal body weight, such as a BMI of twenty-five, in order to turn back or slow down the medical complications of obesity. If you can meet the weight-loss goal you set for yourself in chapter 7 and keep off the weight you have lost, you will go a long way towards improving your health.

Of course, going beyond the goal is fine if the weight is coming off easily. But the reality is that most of us will hit a plateau at some point. If you hit a plateau you cannot break through, accept it and enjoy the weight loss you have already achieved. If you keep pushing harder by starving your body or over-exercising, you risk falling off the wagon and regaining the lost weight. Note that regaining a *few* pounds after reaching your lowest weight is OK—see the box "Have you regained some of your lost weight" in chapter 33.

Some experts prefer to use the waist circumference instead of the BMI as one of the markers of the metabolic syndrome. This is because excess belly fat is the most dangerous fat in the body, and the waist circumference is a better indicator of belly fat than the BMI. However, it is difficult for an untrained person to accurately measure the waist circumference. If you are able to wear pants or dresses you could not get into for years, clearly you are getting rid of belly fat.

Blood pressure: The blood pressure should be no higher than 120/80. The upper number (120) is known as the systolic pressure, and the lower number (80) is known as the diastolic pressure. A person is said to have high blood pressure (hypertension) if either the systolic or diastolic pressure is above normal. In most people with hypertension both the numbers are high.

High blood pressure is called the "silent killer" because it has no symptoms. Unless you actually measure your blood pressure, you have no way of knowing if you have hypertension. Hypertension increases the risk of heart attack, stroke, aortic aneurism, heart failure, and kidney failure.

Obesity greatly increases the risk of developing hypertension. As the weight goes up, the smaller arteries begin to tighten, the kidneys retain salt, and some of the hormones and chemicals produced by the belly fat inflame and damage the walls of the blood vessels. In obese individuals, losing weight usually helps to bring down high blood pressure, but it may not return all the way to normal without the help of medications. This is where your doctor comes in. But you cannot completely turn over the responsibility of checking your blood pressure to your doctor. You need to step in and take charge.

Get a machine and check your blood pressure regularly. Is it staying in the normal range? If it is beginning to creep up, think about what might be causing this. Are you regaining the lost weight? Are you missing doses of your medications? Are you eating too much salt? Is a life situation causing you chronic anxiety? Are you not getting enough sleep? Regardless of the cause, you need to make sure the blood pressure comes down into the normal range. If you can't fix it yourself, talk to your doctor.

If you are on blood pressure medications when you start this program, it is critical you check your blood pressure frequently because it is likely to come down as you lose weight. *In some people the blood pressure begins to drop before there is any weight loss.* So keep an eye on your blood pressure and stay in touch with your doctor in case there is a need to reduce the dose of medications.

Blood Pressure

With every beat, the heart pumps blood into a large artery called the aorta. Arteries that branch off from the aorta channel blood to the brain, arms, abdominal organs, and legs. The walls of these arteries are elastic so they stretch with each heartbeat to accommodate the blood pumped out by the heart. The pressure in these large arteries at the moment they are maximally filled is the systolic pressure.

These large, elastic arteries then squeeze the blood into the smaller arteries that branch through the tissues. As the big arteries empty, the pressure inside them falls. The lowest pressure just before the next heartbeat is the diastolic pressure.

The blood pressure goes up if the heart is pumping faster, as happens when a person is excited, scared, or stressed; from retaining excess salt and water, or if the

arteries, especially the smaller ones, are tighter and narrower than they should be.

Tightening and narrowing of the arteries can be
caused by hormonal effects, by nerve impulses, or
because the arteries have been damaged by inflammation or high blood pressure. Hypertension damages
both large and small arteries, making them stiffer and
narrower. This raises the blood pressure even more, setting up a vicious cycle.

Blood glucose level and hemoglobin A1c: Obesity greatly
increases the risk of diabetes, a condition in which the blood
glucose level is too high. The type of diabetes that is associated with obesity is known as type 2 diabetes. This should not
be confused with type 1 diabetes, which has nothing to do
with obesity.

The complications of diabetes include heart attack, blind-
ness, kidney failure, and damage to nerves and small blood
vessels. Nerve and blood-vessel damage in the lower limbs can
cause ulcers that will not heal, sometimes making it necessary
to amputate a limb.

The blood glucose level depends on many factors: what the
person ate recently, how much insulin is available, and how
well the body cells are responding to insulin. Insulin is made
by the pancreas, an organ tucked behind the stomach. Insulin
helps to keep the blood glucose level in the normal range, and

it also makes sure the body cells are getting the glucose they need for making energy.

As part of keeping the blood glucose level in the normal range, excess glucose is converted into fat. Insulin helps to push this fat into the fat cells for storage. As the cells fill up with fat, they begin to resist the efforts of insulin to push in even more fat, a condition known as insulin resistance. The pancreas attempts to overcome this resistance by making increasing amounts of insulin. For a while it succeeds, but there comes a point at which the insulin resistance cannot be completely overcome and the blood glucose level begins rise above the normal range. The pancreas also sustains damage from being continuously overworked, and this makes the blood glucose level go up even more.

If the person loses weight, the body cells become less insulin resistant and the blood glucose level begins to go down. Whether it comes down all the way or only part way back to normal depends on how healthy the pancreas is and the how much insulin resistance still remains, but any downward trend in the glucose level is a good thing.

The normal blood glucose level after an overnight fast should be between 70 and 100 mg/dl (don't worry about the "mg/dl" part—just remember the numbers). A fasting level from 101 to 125 is known as *impaired glucose tolerance* or *pre-diabetes*. This is an important warning sign, because the risk of progressing to full-fledged diabetes is high. A fasting glucose level of 126 or higher confirms the diagnosis of diabetes.

While measuring the blood glucose level provides useful information, this test can only show what the glucose level was at the moment the blood was drawn. Because the blood glucose level goes up and down all day long, it is useful to know what the *average* level has been in the recent past. This is where the hemoglobin A1c test comes in. This test is also known as the "HbA1c" or "glycated hemoglobin" test.

Understanding the hemoglobin A1c test requires some background knowledge. When a sugar comes in contact with a protein, the sugar chemically alters some of the protein. The higher the sugar level is, the greater the percentage of protein that is altered. This alteration is irreversible; once changed, the protein cannot return to its original form. Hemoglobin is a protein found in red blood cells. The glucose in the blood alters some of the hemoglobin. This altered hemoglobin is known as hemoglobin A1c.

The A1c level depends on the average blood glucose level over the past one to three months. If the blood glucose level has been in the normal range, the hemoglobin A1c level will be 5.6 percent or less. A level of 5.7 to 6.4 percent indicates pre-diabetes; a level of 6.5 percent or higher indicates diabetes. These numbers can vary a little bit depending on how the laboratory does the test. Talk to your doctor about the results and then get a copy for your own records.

To summarize, the blood glucose level tells you what your glucose level was at the moment the blood was drawn, and the A1c level tells you if your average blood glucose level in the past few months has been normal or high. You should try to keep both the fasting blood glucose level and the hemoglobin A1c level in the normal range.

If you have diabetes, you need to monitor your blood glucose level closely when you start this program. *The level can begin to drop even before you lose any weight because of the lower glycemic index of the carbohydrates in your food.* As you lose weight, the blood glucose level is likely to drop even further because of decreasing insulin resistance. Make sure to check with your doctor before starting the program and strictly follow your doctor's instructions about checking your blood glucose level.

Blood cholesterol: "The doctor said that my cholesterol is too high." How often have you heard these words? The cholesterol test or *lipid panel* usually comes back with four numbers: triglycerides, VLDL cholesterol, LDL cholesterol, and HDL cholesterol. What do these numbers mean, and why are they important?

Much of the fat in the body is stored and transported in the form of triglycerides. Triglycerides are used by the body cells as fuel for making energy, and excess triglycerides are stored as fat. Think of triglycerides as the "dollars" of fat currency, to be used or banked. The fat in food is absorbed from the intestine and taken to various parts of the body as triglycerides. The liver also manufactures triglycerides from glucose.

Cholesterol is also a kind of fat, though is more like wax than a typical fat. Cholesterol is used by body cells to keep the cell walls in good repair and to make sex hormones, steroid hormones, and vitamin D. Approximately one-third of the cholesterol in the body comes from the diet and the rest is manufactured internally, mostly by the liver.

Triglycerides and cholesterol are shipped to different parts of the body in the blood. Blood is mostly water, and fat and water do not mix, so the triglycerides and cholesterol have to be packed into special containers before being shipped. These containers are called "lipoproteins." Triglycerides are lighter (less dense) than water, so the more triglyceride that's packed inside a container, the lighter the container is compared to water. Another way of saying this is that the density of the container is lower. VLDL, or Very Low Density Lipoprotein containers are filled with a lot of triglyceride along with some cholesterol. As the triglycerides are dropped off for use by the tissues, the containers change into LDL, or Low Density Lipoprotein.

LDL cholesterol is known as the bad cholesterol. A high level of LDL cholesterol increases the risk of atherosclerosis (hardening of the arteries), heart attack, and stroke. LDL containers can sneak cholesterol under the lining of blood vessels to form little bumps called plaques. As plaques become bigger, they can obstruct the flow of blood. If the blood vessel is in a critical organ such as the heart, the reduction in blood flow can lead to angina. If a plaque ruptures, a blood clot can form at the site; the result is a heart attack or stroke.

In people who have previously had a heart attack, lowering the LDL cholesterol level reduces the risk of subsequent heart attacks. Lowering the LDL level in diabetics also reduces the risk of a first heart attack. Even in people without diabetes, lowering the LDL cholesterol level provides protection against heart attack, especially if there are other risk factors present such as obesity, high blood pressure, smoking, or a family history of heart attack at an early age (younger than 55 years in men or 65 years in women).

It is important to keep the LDL level within the recommended guidelines. These guidelines depend on the person's

medical history. Talk to your doctor to find out what the recommended guidelines are for you. Losing weight and eating a
healthy diet will often help to lower the LDL level, but in many
people this is not enough. Fortunately, there are effective medications to help lower the LDL level; your doctor will guide you.

As with LDL cholesterol, there is evidence that a high level
of triglycerides and VLDL cholesterol can also damage blood
vessel walls and increase the risk of heart attack, although the
connection is not as clear as it is for LDL cholesterol. In addition, a high triglyceride level tends to lower the level of good
cholesterol (see below).

A high triglyceride level is often an indicator the diet needs
attention—there is too much high-glycemic carbohydrate in
the diet. The triglyceride level is also high in people with diabetes if the disease is not under good control. Drinking alcohol
also raises the triglyceride level.

Reducing high-glycemic carbohydrates in the diet, which
you are already doing, will help lower the triglyceride level.
Exercise and fish oil also help. In extreme cases, your doctor
can prescribe medications to lower the triglyceride level.

Finally, there is HDL cholesterol. HDL stands for High
Density Lipoprotein. Empty HDL containers are made in the
liver and sent off around the body to collect excess cholesterol
(including the cholesterol in the walls of the arteries) and
bring it back to the liver for disposal.

HDL cholesterol is called the good cholesterol precisely
because HDL containers collect and remove excess cholesterol
from the body, so having a higher level of HDL cholesterol is
protective. A level of more than 60 mg/dl lowers the risk of

heart attack and stroke; conversely, a level less than 50 mg/dl in women and 40 mg/dl in men increases this risk.

Exercise helps to raise the HDL cholesterol level, as does reducing high-glycemic carbohydrates in the diet because this reduces the triglyceride level. Moderate alcohol consumption also increases the HDL level. Stopping smoking and taking fish oil supplements will help raise the HDL level. In certain situations, your doctor might prescribe medications to try and increase the HDL level.

In addition to the diet, genetic factors play an important role in determining the triglyceride and cholesterol levels. While weight loss, eating a healthy diet, and moderate exercise certainly help in improving the numbers, these lifestyle changes cannot always overcome a strong underlying genetic tendency. This is one reason why medications are often necessary for proper cholesterol management. So get your cholesterol levels checked and work with your doctor to achieve the best possible cholesterol profile.

Doctor Alok says:

- The biggest reward of weight loss is better health for the rest of your life.
- Obesity, along with high blood pressure, a high blood sugar level, a high blood triglyceride level, and a low blood level of good cholesterol are warning signs of health problems in the future.
- Even if only one of these is present, there is cause for concern.

- If three are present at the same time—that's a huge red flag called the metabolic syndrome.
- Keep an eye on your weight, check your blood pressure regularly, understand what the blood tests mean, and work with your doctor to keep the numbers as normal as possible.

Chapter 35

Keeping the Right State of Mind

Managing one's weight is so much easier when the mind is calm and life seems to be under control. Stress and worry are enemies of healthy eating and weight management. Unfortunately, stress is a part of life.

Stress is a reaction to adverse life events and the future possibility of such events. Some of these events are out of our control, but small changes in how we live and look at life can help reduce that out-of-control feeling and bring down the stress level. Below are five life lessons that have helped me.

I Make Lists

I keep a written to-do list and prioritize the tasks. Without a list, there is a constant, nagging worry in the back of my mind that I am forgetting something. This worry drains my energy and adds to my stress.

A list can be kept on a cell phone or computer, but I find that a handwritten list on a 3" X 5" card works best for me because physically crossing off a completed task is very satisfying. I add new tasks to my list as they come up, and every few days I transfer the leftover tasks to a fresh card. As I do so, I re-prioritize the tasks if necessary.

I identify the tasks I want to avoid and do these first. I have a tendency to procrastinate, filling my time with minor and less important activities while putting off difficult or stressful tasks even if they are more important. Listing the tasks I would normally avoid and taking care of them first gives me a sense of achievement. The better I feel about myself, the more energy I have to make good eating choices.

If I am going through an unusually busy or stressful time in my life, I keep an additional card and pencil at the bedside. If I wake up in the middle of the night with a sudden recollection of something that needs to be done, I write it down on the card. Then I am able to go back to sleep because I've released the task from my mind.

So if you don't regularly make and use to-do lists, give it a try.

I Have Learned to Say No to Protect My Time

Saying no can be difficult, but it can also be liberating.

When asked to take on yet another responsibility, we do not always have the choice to refuse. But sometimes we do, and learning to occasionally say no gently but firmly is an important part of keeping one's life under control.

It is possible to become addicted to the gratitude of others, of wanting to be perceived as always being helpful. "Mary is so nice— she never says no." If Mary can handle all her responsibilities and still have time for herself, good for her. But if Mary is putting on a brave face while running herself ragged—well, that is not so good.

Sometimes we can't even say no to ourselves. We schedule our time too tightly; we try to do too many things. Some of us are extremely driven in our professional lives and try to accomplish too much. But there has to be a balance between accomplishment and health. What is the point of laboring so hard that we ruin our health and are not around to enjoy the fruits of our labor?

We all need some down time. Learn to occasionally say no to give your mind and body a chance to relax and restore.

I Play to My Strengths

As far as possible, I try to take on tasks that match my skills, tasks that I enjoy doing and can do well. Taking on responsibilities for which I am temperamentally unsuited or need skills I do not possess (or cannot obtain) is stressful for me.

Playing to one's strengths takes less time and energy than compensating for one's weaknesses. We need to know who we are, how we like to approach tasks, what we do well. Some of us do our best work if assigned a job and left alone; others function well in a group. Some are good at handling short-term projects; others can take on a long-term responsibility, staying with it month after month and year after year. Some are comfortable at taking risks; others are risk-averse. Some are natural leaders; others prefer to follow a good leader.

There is no right or wrong way to be because the world needs all of us. The question *you* have to ask is—who am I? Do

I know my strengths and weaknesses? Do I know what I do well and what stresses me out?

These are important questions. In your professional life, choosing your tasks and responsibilities wisely will help you succeed because you will accomplish more, and in less time. In your social life—your club, your church, or hobby group— you need to be selective about when to volunteer and when to politely decline. You have to be able to say, "This is not something I can do well." You will use your time and energy more effectively, you will have less stress in your life, and your body will thank you.

I Find it Useful to Say, "Let's See What Happens Next!"

When something consequential happens in life, it is normal to feel happy or sad, exhilarated or depressed. But before I get too emotionally wrapped up in an event, I have learned to reflect on the reality that *no event occurs in isolation*. Events have consequences, which in turn have other consequences—and the consequences are unpredictable.

Every event in your life and mine is just one link in a never-ending chain of events. Every event, without exception, influences future events in unpredictable ways. While I might feel happy or sad about something that has just happened, I don't really know what this event will lead to. A seeming misfortune sometimes turns out to be a blessing in disguise; the loss of a job can force one to finally go find a better one. The opposite is just as true. Not all lottery winners end up happy; some see their lives fall apart.

Stepping back and taking the long view, looking at an event as just one link in a never-ending chain of events, helps me deal with the ups and downs, the fortunes and misfortunes of life, with more equanimity.

There is a Chinese parable about an old farmer. This farmer had a small plot of land that his son helped him till and plant, and a horse that pulled his wagon to the market so he could sell his crops.

One day, the horse ran away into the forest. The farmer's neighbor came over to sympathize. "Poor you," said the neighbor, "now you can't take your crop to the market to sell. How are you going to make any money?" The farmer just smiled and said, "Let's see what happens next."

A day later the horse came back, bringing two wild horses with him. The neighbor came over to celebrate. "You now have three horses! The gods are smiling on you! You are the most fortunate man in the village!" The farmer just smiled. "Let's see what happens next," he said.

The next day the farmer's son was trying to tame one of the wild horses. The horse threw him, and the son broke his leg. The neighbor came over to sympathize. "You poor man," said the neighbor. "Now you have no one to help you till the field and plant the crops. How will you grow anything?" The farmer just smiled. "Let's see what happens next," he said.

The next day, the king's soldiers came to the village looking for conscripts for the king's army. All the young men in the village were taken away except the farmer's son, because he had a broken leg.

Now was that bad luck? Good luck? It depends on what happens next.

Like the Chinese farmer, I can smile and say, "Let's see what happens next!" And anytime you can smile instead of stressing yourself out, you will make better eating choices.

I Have Learned to Actively Seek Happiness Instead of Waiting for Happiness to Come to Me

In today's food environment, weight management requires making eating choices that go against the deeply ingrained instinct to make and store fat. This tension between what I want to do and what my body wants to do is a constant backdrop to all weight-loss efforts.

Going against instinct consumes a lot of energy. This energy has to be periodically restored, just as a drained battery has to be recharged. Nothing recharges me as effectively as being deeply, truly, happy.

True happiness is different from pleasure. Pleasure is superficial and transient. Seeing an enjoyable movie, partying with friends, or reading a good book gives me pleasure, but that pleasure begins to fade as soon as the pleasurable experience is over. Pleasure is an important part of life, but pleasure alone is not sufficient to adequately recharge the battery. For this we need happiness. *Happiness reaches deep into the psyche and changes one's outlook on life.* To a happy person, the world seems a better place.

One source of happiness is achievement, the sense of satisfaction that comes from successfully accomplishing a difficult task. The task can relate to the external world, such as achieving a sales goal, rendering an unsatisfied customer happy, making an important research discovery in the laboratory, learning to sew, or teaching your child to ride a bicycle. The task can also be internal, such as reaching your weight-loss target.

But accomplishments don't come by every day. Fortunately, there is second source of happiness out there for the taking, a source that never runs dry. This is the happiness that comes from doing something for others without expectation of reward, from the unselfish giving of one's time, energy, or talent. Look around you, at your family, your friends, your co-workers. Can you do something for them that would make their lives, or even just their day, a little better? Then do it, but do it without expecting anything in return. Your happiness will be its own reward.

Also look outside your circle. Think about volunteering for a good cause. Volunteering means more than just writing a check for charity or donating a few cans of food. The kind of volunteering that recharges the batteries requires actually showing up and doing something. Helping serve food to the needy, tutoring a student who needs a little help, reading to seniors in an old folk's home—these are the activities that will make you truly happy. And the happier you are, the more easily you will be able to keep off the weight you have lost. Opportunities for volunteering are everywhere. Find some in your community, show up, and give a little of yourself.

There is no limit to the supply of happiness. Go get your share.

Be happy.

Doctor Alok says:

- Stress is the enemy of weight loss; happiness is the friend of weight loss. Learn to avoid stress and seek happiness.
- Make to-do lists so you can stop stressing about what you might have forgotten.
- Learn to say no to protect your time.
- Go with your strengths.
- Remember that everything in life leads to something else. Don't get too hung up on what happens today.
- Actively seek happiness. Volunteer for something worthwhile.

Part 7:
More Useful Stuff

This section has four chapters.

Chapter 36 adds to your knowledge of food chemistry and physiology. The more educated you are as a consumer of food, the better you will be able to look after your body.

Chapter 37 is a guide to almost every type of food, from beverages (including alcohol) to dessert. Is coffee good or bad for you? Which vegetables should you eat in abundance, and which should be eaten in moderation? Are some fruits better for you than others? Meat, grains, dairy, nuts, oils, desserts—it's all there.

Chapter 38 expands your recipe options. Once you have completed the first two weeks of the program, you can use this chapter to start adding to your repertoire of recipes. These recipes have been designed for you by a professional chef. Each dinner recipe serves two to three people, and the leftovers can become the next day's lunch for one person.

Finally, chapter 39 brings you a variety of salads (and dressings)—leaf salads, vegetables, beans, fruits, cheese, and proteins. You will do yourself a lot of good if, on most days, one of your major meals is colorful salad. But eating the same salad day after day can become boring. This chapter offers pointers on how to keep your salads always fresh and attractive by using different combinations of ingredients.

Chapter 36

The Least You Need to Know
About Nutrition

Food has two major components: macronutrients and micronutrients. The terms are self-explanatory—we need macronutrients in relatively large amounts and micronutrients in smaller (micro) amounts.

Macronutrients

Water: Water is the most important macronutrient. A person can live for weeks without food but only for a few days without water. An adult needs to drink about four pints of water a day, but can survive on half that amount (though it won't be pleasant). At the other extreme, drinking eight or ten pints a day won't hurt; the body just gets rid of the excess in the urine. Of course, a person who is exercising vigorously or spending time outdoors in the hot sun will need more than the basic four pints.

You don't need to worry about whether you are getting enough water. The body is very sensitive to a shortage of water and will make you thirsty to ensure you restock when necessary.

You also do not need to drink extra water to flush out the system. As long as a person is not dehydrated, the body is very efficient at clearing out its wastes in the normal amount of urine.

The bottom line: Respect thirst. As long as you drink water whenever you feel thirsty, your body is getting enough water. Also, you don't need oxygenated water, spring water, vitamin-enriched water, or flavored water. Just regular old water is fine. Don't waste your money on improved water. Spend it on fresh, natural *food* instead.

Fiber: Even though we cannot digest and absorb the fiber in our food, it plays a critical role in keeping us healthy.

There are two kinds of fiber—insoluble fiber and soluble fiber. Insoluble fiber does not dissolve in water. Insoluble fiber is the crunch in leaves and roots and stems and fruits. The bran that forms the thick outer shell of beans and grains is also insoluble fiber.

Insoluble fiber has at least four major functions. First, it makes chewing necessary, so it takes longer to eat a meal. This allows the body to reduce hunger as the stomach is gradually filling up. Processed, fiber-free food requires less chewing so it goes in too fast, making it easy to over-shoot hunger and eat excessively.

Second, insoluble fiber provides a feeling of fullness, which also discourages over-eating. Thirdly, the insoluble fiber "cage" protects food from being digested too rapidly by serving as a physical barrier between the food and the digestive enzymes (see chapter 9). This ensures that nutrients are absorbed at a slow enough pace for the body to handle them properly, sending each where it is needed—a process that is critical for good health. Finally, insoluble fiber provides bulk and solidity to the intestinal contents. This keeps things moving and avoids constipation. This, in turn, reduces the risk of appendicitis, diverticulosis, and perhaps even colon cancer.

Soluble fiber is found in beans (pinto, garbanzo, black, red, etc.) and lentils; oats (but not in most other grains); fruits such as prunes, apple, pears, and bananas; and in psyllium husk. Soluble fiber dissolves in water and swells up like an invisible sponge. This sponge can mop up glucose and slow down its rate of absorption, in essence lowering the glycemic index of the meal as a whole (see chapter 9). Soluble fiber also binds to cholesterol and prevents it from being absorbed, which is why oat cereal is touted as being able to lower the blood cholesterol level. Finally, soluble fiber helps to maintain a thriving population of bacteria in the colon, which is also important for good health.

A diet that is rich in natural vegetables, fruits, and beans provides all the fiber a person needs.

Protein: Proteins are the bricks and mortar with which we build tissues and organs. Proteins are found in meat and milk, beans and legumes and lentils, and to a smaller extent, in grains and vegetables.

Proteins are made of building blocks called amino-acids. Humans need twenty-one different kinds of amino acids. Twelve of the twenty-one we can make in the body, but the other nine have to come from our food. These nine are called *essential* amino acids. Proteins in meat, milk, and eggs contain all the essential amino acids. Most vegetable proteins contain some but not all. Eating a variety of plant foods ensures that we get all the essential amino acids—some from one food, and some from another. Soy protein and quinoa are two plant products that contain all of the essential amino acids.

Unless a person is eating a very restrictive diet, there is no need to worry about getting enough protein. In fact, the western diet today probably has too much protein. Excess protein tends to acidify the blood and can, at least in theory, increase the risk of osteoporosis and fractures by leaching out calcium from the bones. So go easy on the meat; eat beans in moderation, and fill up on veggies and fruits.

From the weight management perspective, protein is a non-issue. Any excess of protein in the diet is eliminated in the urine. While some of the amino acids in proteins can be converted into glucose if necessary and used as fuel, glucose is not manufactured from amino acids just to be turned into fat and stored.

Carbohydrates: Digestible carbohydrates—starch and sugar—are one of the two fuels used by the body, fat being the other.

Starch has been the major food for most humans since times immemorial. Starch, as we already know from chapter 9, is a long chain of glucose particles linked to each other. In addition to glucose, there are many other types of sugar in our food. Fructose or "fruit sugar" is found in fruits along with glucose. Fructose is much sweeter than glucose; agave nectar is almost pure fructose. Glucose and fructose link up to form table sugar, or sucrose. Milk contains a sugar called lactose, in which glucose is linked to another sugar known as galactose.

Glucose is a major fuel for the body, but all these sugars can be used as a fuel source and all can be turned into fat. Just because a food has a low glycemic index does not mean it has no sugar because the glycemic index applies only to foods that contain glucose. The food may well contain other types of sugars. Always look for the total sugar on the label.

Fat: In addition to glucose, fat is the other major fuel used by the body for producing energy. Dietary fat comes in two forms, saturated and unsaturated. Saturation refers to how many of available carbon atom bonds in the fat have a hydrogen atom attached. If all available bonds are occupied, the fat is saturated with hydrogen; if not, the fat is unsaturated. Unsaturated fats are further divided into mono- or poly-unsaturated, depending on the chemical structure.

Saturated fat is solid at room temperature. All animal fat—chicken fat, beef tallow, and even the fat in fish—is mostly saturated fat, which is why animal fat is solid. But animal fat does contain some unsaturated fat, and this will become important when we get to omega-3 and omega-6 fatty acids.

Unsaturated fats are liquid at room temperature; we call them oils. Most vegetable fats are unsaturated. Seed oils such as canola oil and soybean oil tend to be poly-unsaturated, while olive oil, which is extracted mostly from the pulp of the olive, is largely mono-unsaturated. The only two vegetable fats that have a high proportion of saturated fat are coconut oil and palm oil (also known as red palm oil), and both of these are solid at room temperature.

Eating an excess of saturated fat has been linked to an increase in bad cholesterol and heart disease. However, the link is not entirely clear. The effects of saturated fat may also have to do with whether the meat comes from grass-fed animals (better) or corn-fed animals (not so good). That said, most of the animal fat available today is from corn-fed animals. Unsaturated fats, in general, seem to be heart-neutral or even a little bit heart-healthy.

Omega-3 and omega-6 fats: Fat is made up of building blocks called fatty acids. Some of these can be manufactured in the body, but others can only be obtained from the diet. These are known as essential fatty acids. Omega-3 and omega-6 fatty acids are examples of essential fatty acids. While the role of omega-3 and omega-6 fatty acids in human health and disease is not clear, there are some theoretical considerations worth noting.

Some types of omega-6 fatty acids promote inflammation. While inflammation is a normal and necessary component of a competent immune system, an excess of dietary omega-6 fats may lead to excessive and inappropriate inflammation and worsen conditions that have a background of inflammation such as atherosclerosis, asthma, and arthritis.

Omega-3 fatty acids are anti-inflammatory and anti-clotting. These fatty acids balance the effects of omega-6 fatty acids. To remain in good health, the diet needs to contain both omega-6 and omega-3 fatty acids in an approximate ratio of 4:1. In general, omega-6 fatty acids are found in seeds and nuts (with some notable exceptions such as flax and chia seeds and walnuts—these have a good amount of omega-3). Omega-3 fatty acids, in addition to deep-sea cold-water fish, are found in green vegetables. Eating food that has an abundance of green, and eating the meat of animals that are raised on grass, should provide an adequate amount of omega-3 fatty acids.

Unfortunately, the ratio of omega-6 to omega-3 in the American diet in now more like 10:1; some estimations place it as high as 30:1. This is because of the tremendous increase of corn and soybean products in the food chain, and this includes the meat of corn-fed animals. It now appears difficult for us to get enough omega-3 from dietary sources to counteract the effects of the omega-6 fatty acids.

One rich source of omega-3 fatty acids is the ocean. Green marine algae produce omega-3 fatty acids. Fish concentrate these healthy fats in their tissues. Salt-water fish that live in cold water, such as salmon, anchovies, and herring are particularly high in omega-3 fats. Omega-3 fats are also available in fish-oil supplements. Vegetarians have the choice of flax seed oil or oil obtained from marine algae. The latter might be better choice because this type of omega-3 can be used directly by the body, while the omega-3 in flax seed oil first has to be converted into the active form and the efficiency of this conversion is unpredictable.

Trans-fats: These are produced when vegetable oils are solidified into margarine or shortening by saturating them with hydrogen (see above). Trans-fats are found only in miniscule amounts in nature and the body does not seem to know how to deal with them—another example of altered foods that confuse the body. Trans-fats increase the risk of heart attacks, more so than even saturated fats. Current standards in the

USA allow foods with a small amount of trans-fats per serving to be labeled as trans-fat free; some margarines, for example, carry this labeling—but why take a chance? If you are using margarine on your bread, use real butter instead.

Micronutrients

Salt: We need less salt than you might think. A person in good health with normal kidney function can live on as little as a fifth of a teaspoonful a day. Hunter-gatherers who lived far from the ocean probably did not eat salt other than what was naturally present in food. Of course, now we expect our food to be salted to taste, and that's OK; unless there is a medical reason for doing so, there is no need to tightly restrict salt intake. But there is also no reason to eat an excess of a substance that we are not designed to eat in excess.

Food labels provide the sodium content of the food in "mg" or "milligrams." Current dietary guidelines recommend eating no more than 2000 mg of sodium daily. This includes sodium from all sources—salt added to food and salt in preserved meats, cheese, pickles, canned food, chips, and salted nuts, and everything else. It is important to read labels.

Table salt is two-fifths sodium by weight, so 2000 mg of sodium is equal to 5000 mg of table salt, or about one teaspoonful. If you prepare most of your food from fresh ingredients, one teaspoon of salt is a reasonable daily limit to aim for.

Vitamins and minerals: Humans did quite well for a long time without knowing anything about vitamins and minerals. That is the whole point of micronutrients—we need so little of these that a natural, balanced diet takes care of the body's need without us even thinking about it. Vitamin deficiency diseases are a by-product of an unnatural or unbalanced diet. Scurvy, caused by vitamin C deficiency, was rampant in sailors who lived for months at a time on hardtack biscuits and preserved meats with no fresh fruits or vegetables. Just a little bit of lime juice in the diet took care of the scurvy, which is why British sailors were called "limeys." Similarly, pellagra, caused by deficiency of the vitamin niacin, was widespread in populations that depended on corn for a majority of their nutritional needs.

If you are eating a diet that is rich in colorful, natural foods, you should not have to worry about vitamins and minerals. However, our modern fast-paced life puts unusual stresses and strains on the body, and stress can increase the need for vitamins. We also don't live "naturally"—for example, many of us spend hardly any time in direct (not through glass) sunlight that is so essential for making vitamin D. For these reasons, it might not be a bad idea to take a multivitamin and mineral pill a few times a week. I am making this recommendation with some hesitation because there is no good evidence to back it up.

Vegans, of course, need to take a vitamin B12 supplement because there is no vitamin B12 in plants. This vitamin is found only in animal products.

Phytochemicals and anti-oxidants: Phytochemicals are naturally occurring colorful compounds found in plants. These compounds may have anti-cancer and anti-inflammatory properties and also play a beneficial role in people with diabetes and heart disease. Anti-oxidants are a sub-group of phytochemicals that neutralize harmful oxygen radicals (also known as free radicals) formed in the body in the course of normal metabolism. Oxygen radicals have been implicated in conditions such as wrinkling of the skin with age, Alzheimer's disease, and atherosclerosis. Berries are rich in anti-oxidants, and so are other colorful fruits and vegetables. Red wine, green tea, spices such as cumin, coriander, and cinnamon, as well as dark chocolate are also good sources of anti-oxidants.

Most of the evidence for the benefits of phytochemicals and anti-oxidants has come from animal experiments. A number of trials in humans are ongoing. One unexpected result is that taking a large amount of a *single* anti-oxidant such as beta-carotene or vitamin E as a pill does not reduce the risk of cancer or cardiovascular disease. In fact, high dose supplementation of a single anti-oxidant may actually increase the risk of some types of cancers.

It makes sense to accept that nature intended for us to eat a *mixture* of fresh fruits and vegetables. As far as food is concerned, it is almost impossible to improve on nature, so the value of concentrated anti-oxidant supplements or expensive bottled anti-oxidant juices is questionable. Eating plenty of natural, colorful fruits and vegetables gives us all the phytochemicals and anti-oxidants we need.

Chapter 37

Food Choices after the
First Two Weeks

Beverages

Coffee: The medical literature is full of mixed messages for and against coffee. The bottom line seems to be that having a couple of cups of coffee in the morning and another in the afternoon is just fine—but limit the amount of cream and sugar. One tablespoon of half-and-half contains twenty calories, and two teaspoons of sugar add about forty more. If you load your coffee three times a day with cream and sugar, you are not doing yourself any favors.

Also, having sugar thrice daily may keep your sugar addiction going. So have your coffee black, or with as little milk and sugar as you can get away with. What about using sugar substitutes in your coffee? See below.

Diet drinks and sugar substitutes: Diet drinks may be an example of something that looks good on paper but is not so good in real life. Some studies have actually associated diet drinks with weight gain. The reason for this is not clear. It may be that people who are gaining weight anyhow tend to switch

221

to diet drinks; it may be that the sweet taste of diet drinks triggers the appetite and keeps the sugar addiction going, just like real sugar; it may be that sugar substitutes, because of their sweet taste, fool the body into making insulin—but with no sugar coming, the unnecessary insulin just lowers the blood sugar level and increases hunger. Whatever the reason, diet drinks do not seem to be a good substitute for sugared drinks. Avoid both.

Also, sugar substitutes are chemicals that have no normal function in the body. Even if these are presumed to be safe, why load your body with unnecessary chemicals?

Fruit juice and fruit drinks: This is just sugar water loaded with empty calories. Drinking a glass of apple juice fills up your body with the sugar from four apples with none of the fiber. Avoid fruit juice. If you want fruit, eat the whole fruit.

So what should you drink? The same thing our ancestors drank for thousands of years, the same thing every other animal drinks: water.

Vegetables

Here are some general rules:

Any part of the plant that grows above the ground and is called a vegetable can be eaten without restriction. These include leaves (e.g., lettuce, spinach, cabbage), fruits that are called vegetables (tomatoes, peppers, eggplants), and shoots (asparagus, celery). All these are full of fiber and have very little starch and sugar. The only exceptions are corn and peas (but not snap peas); these are high in starch and should be used sparingly.

When you leave the produce section of your supermarket (or the local farmers co-op), your shopping basket should have a rainbow of colors in it. Leaves, fruits, and shoots are full of vitamins, minerals, and anti-oxidants. As a general rule, the more colorful the vegetable the more the micronutrients it contains. For example, red and orange vegetables and fruits have carotene, from which we make vitamin A; purple ones have flavonoids, which are anti-oxidants; and dark green ones have iron and calcium.

Root vegetables are another matter. Many root vegetables contain useful micronutrients, but all root vegetables are starchy. Just as animals store excess glucose as fat, many plants store glucose in their roots as starch. For root vegetables, use the following rules:

Potatoes: These tend to be very high in starch. Eat them only on freestyling days and use small red potatoes or new potatoes. Leave the skin on because it contains fiber. Avoid large mealy potatoes.

Carrots, sweet potatoes: Eat these, but in moderation. These do have starch, but they also have useful micronutrients.

Radishes, onions, turnips, beets: Use these as an ingredient in salads, sauces, and gravies.

Fruits

You should have one to two servings (total) of any of the following daily:

- *Berries,* such as strawberries (5), blueberries (1/2 cup)
- *Crunchy fruits,* such as an apple or pear (each is one serving)

- *Pitted fruits*, such as plums, nectarines, and apricots (each is one serving)
- *Citrus fruits*, such as orange (each is one serving) or grapefruit (½ is one serving)

Juicy fruits and soft fruits, such as watermelon, grapes, pineapple, and ripe bananas are high in sugar. Eat these only occasionally, and no more than 1/2 a cup in a day.

Do not liquefy your fruits in a blender. Not only will you destroy the fiber cage (which will allow the sugar to be absorbed very quickly), you are also likely to drink more fruits at one sitting than you will ever eat at one time. How often do you eat an apple *and* a banana *and* an orange *and* a handful of blueberries all at once? But it is easy to throw these into a blender all together and drink them. That's a lot of sugar.

Grain

Sprouted-grain products (such as Ezekiel 4:9 bread, tortillas, pita, pasta) are recommended, up to a maximum of 225 "grain" calories a day. *Note: If you have a gluten allergy, you should not use any product with wheat, spelt (a type of wheat), barley, or rye. Talk to your doctor about foods that are suitable for you.*

Whole grain **bread**, tortillas, pita, and pasta are acceptable if you cannot find sprouted grain products. Look for "100 percent whole grain" or "100 percent whole wheat" on the label. Also, if a product advertised as whole grain is silky-smooth to the touch and tastes just like a white-flour product, the grain has been ground too fine and the fiber cage has been completely pulverized. Avoid such products.

Quinoa (pronounced "keen-wa") is a great substitute for rice. It is the seed of a plant from the Andes Mountains in South America. Quinoa was used as food by the Incas for thousands of years. It has high protein content and is one of the few vegetarian foods to contain all the essential amino acids. Quinoa, as it comes from the wild, has a slight bitter coating and needs to be rinsed once with water. Most of the quinoa sold today is pre-rinsed; even so, it is not a bad idea to rinse it, just in case. Quinoa floats in water and has to be drained carefully after rinsing. Quinoa is now readily available in the United States. It comes as red or white quinoa. You can use either.

Do not use corn products as a substitute for grain. These products are often made from processed corn flour and have a high glycemic index.

Legumes and Lentils

All beans (including garbanzo beans) and lentils are fine. It is best to use beans and lentils with the skin on. Washed or skinless beans are also available in Indian grocery stores. These can be used but contain less fiber.

Dairy

Milk is not a natural food for humans after infancy and is not necessary for good health if the diet is otherwise adequate. A glass of whole milk has 140 calories and glass of skim milk has 80 calories. There is no reason to ingest unnecessary calories. If you must have milk, use skim milk. Plain, unsweetened soy milk is an acceptable substitute because it has less carbohydrate—but it, too, is an artificial food. Avoid whole milk except for little bit in coffee or tea. If you want to increase your calcium intake, taking a pill instead of drinking milk will save you the calories.

Hard cheese such as cheddar can be used in moderation, up to two ounces daily in salads and snacks. Cheese is high in calories and fat, but in this program cheese is used mainly as a preventer—hard cheese has a satisfying mouth-feel and is very effective in taking the edge off your hunger, and this prevents you from eating foods that are nutritionally worse than cheese.

Feta cheese can be used in salads.

Unsweetened, plain yogurt can be used in moderation.

Meat and eggs

Eggs: There are no definite recommendations on egg consumption. Up to one egg daily appears to be acceptable if your cholesterol level is normal. However, if you have a high cholesterol level, restrict eggs to two to three times per week and talk to your doctor. You can use additional egg white, as much as you want. Look for a farmers market in your area and use eggs from free-range chickens if possible.

Poultry: Use white meat of chicken and turkey with the skin removed. Limit dark meat because it contains saturated fats. If you must use roasted chicken and turkey breast from the deli, try to get the reduced sodium variety. Free-range chickens are available, but tend to be quite expensive.

Fish: Salmon is a good source of omega-3 fatty acids. Buy wild-caught salmon if available. The quality of farm-raised salmon appears to vary from producer to producer, and farm-raised fish may have less omega-3 and more bad fats than wild-caught fish. There is also concern about contamination with PCBs; however, the evidence against eating farm-raised salmon is not strong at this time.

Sardines are another good source of omega-3 fatty acids. Tuna is also a good source of omega-3s, but should be eaten in moderation because of potential mercury contamination. There are specific guidelines concerning the intake of tuna and other fish for children and pregnant women at **http://www.epa.gov/waterscience/fishadvice/advice.html**.

Any other fish, fresh or frozen, is fine. However, if you are looking for omega-3 fatty acids, tilapia (which is always farm-raised when sold commercially) and farm-raised catfish are not good sources.

Shrimp are allowed, especially if you can find shrimp caught in your local waters. Bagged, frozen shrimp are typically farm-raised.

Beef: Use lean cuts in limited amounts. Use grass-fed beef if possible; it has less fat and may be more heart-healthy—but it is expensive. Bison in the United States are now mostly corn-fed, so bison meat (unless specifically labeled as grass-fed) would seem to have little if any advantage over beef.

Pork: Use lean cuts in limited amounts.

Processed meats such as bacon, salami, bologna, hot dogs and frankfurters, pastrami, etc. should be avoided except as an occasional treat—too many chemicals, too much salt.

Nuts and Seeds

Walnuts and almonds have heart-healthy fats. But they are also packed with calories; eat no more than twenty almonds or ten walnut halves a day except in special circumstances (see the sections on business travel and vacations). The nuts should not be roasted or salted.

Flax, pumpkin, and sunflower seeds, up to a tablespoonful a day, are also allowed.

Peanut butter can be used in moderation. One tablespoonful has about one hundred calories. If you use natural peanut butter, it tends to separate out into oil and solids and can make a mess when you mix it. Keep the bottle upside down for a day before stirring—now the oil will be at the bottom and won't splash. If your grocery store has a machine for making fresh peanut butter on the spot, use it. This way you know what's going into the peanut butter.

Peanuts and cashews are usually salted and easy to overeat. These, along with *macadamia* nuts, also contain too much fat. Avoid them.

Fats

Use no more than three tablespoonsful of oil daily (1-1/2 ounces). Extra virgin olive oil is good for use as salad dressing and for light sautéing. Canola oil is recommended for higher-heat cooking. It has a better omega-3 to omega-6 ratio than other seed oils.

If you use butter on your toast, reduce the oil quota for the day. Avoid other animal fats. Avoid trans-fats.

Suggestions for Dessert

Try any one of the following:
* *Fruit:* a couple of strawberries, a small handful of grapes, half an apple

- *Chocolate:* One square of 70 percent chocolate
- *Nuts:* up to twenty almonds or ten walnut halves (if not consumed earlier in the day)
- *Wine:* two ounces (see below)

Alcohol

You should not use any alcohol during the first two weeks of the program. After that, you can have half a glass of wine with supper, if you must. You can have more on freestyling days. See chapter 27 for more information on alcohol intake. But if you are having difficulty losing weight, cut out the alcohol.

Chapter 38

Recipe Suggestions After the First Two Weeks

This section has ten fill-up/tune-up meal combinations. The leftovers from the fill-up meal are used to supplement the tune-up meal that follows.

After you have finished the first two weeks of the program, you should start adding some of these recipes to your eating plan. These tasty recipes have been designed by a professional chef to be within the program guidelines. Some of the recipes might stretch your culinary abilities, but learning to cook good-tasting, healthy food is an important part of long-term weight management. It prevents boredom and reduces the risk of straying from the program.

The fill-up meal recipes will take care of the meat and the starch part of the plate. You will have to add vegetables of your choice to complete the plate. Use your imagination—you can supplement the meal with grilled or roasted vegetables (as you have learned to do in the past two weeks), or make a small side-salad (see also chapter 39), or just cut up some tomatoes, cucumbers, apples, etc., or even microwave a frozen vegetable mix. If you like greens such as spinach or kale, you can do a quick sauté and add these to your plate.

1A: Chicken in Wine
Serves 2-3

1 ½ cups dry quinoa
3 cups water
3 chicken breast halves, each about the size of a deck of cards
1 teaspoon all-purpose seasoning blend (recipe towards end of chapter)
1 tablespoon canola oil
¼ cup sliced shallots or onion
½ pear (sliced)
½ cup white wine
3 sprigs of fresh thyme
2 tablespoons shredded parmesan cheese

1. Bring quinoa and water to boil, stir, cover, and reduce heat to low. Simmer for 15-20 minutes. Let set for 5 minutes, uncovered, off heat, then fluff. Alternatively, you may use a rice cooker using the same proportions of quinoa and water. Reserve 1 cup cooked quinoa for tomorrow's lunch.
2. If the chicken breast is thick, slice into two pieces horizontally. Season the chicken and place in skillet with heated canola oil. Cook 5 minutes per side or until cooked through. Remove from skillet and set aside. Reserve 1 chicken breast for tomorrow's lunch.

3. Sauté shallots in the same skillet for 5 minutes or until lightly browned. Add pears, wine, and thyme along with cooked chicken. Cover and reduce heat to simmer for 5 minutes. Serve chicken atop cooked quinoa.

1B: Quinoa Chicken Salad
Serves 1

1 ½ cups chopped fresh vegetables such as broccoli, cucumber, mushrooms
1 cup cooked quinoa
1 cooked diced chicken breast
2 tablespoons diced red bell pepper
1 tablespoon dried cranberries
2 tablespoons sliced green onions
2 tablespoons chopped walnuts
2 tablespoons Lemon-thyme Vinaigrette (recipe towards end of chapter)

Stir together all ingredients. Chill overnight.

2A: Grilled Salmon
Serves 2-3

3 salmon fillets about the size of your palm (snapper or halibut may be substituted)
½ teaspoon all-purpose seasoning blend (recipe towards end of chapter)
½ teaspoon nutmeg

1 teaspoon chopped fresh ginger

2 tablespoons apple cider vinegar

1 tablespoon olive oil

1 clove chopped garlic

1 cup dry lentils

1 tablespoon canola oil

½ cup sliced shallot or onion

2 tablespoons chopped dried apricots

½ teaspoon salt

1. Combine the spices, vinegar, and olive oil and marinate the salmon, preferably overnight. Grill or broil on medium heat for 10-12 minutes until fish barely flakes. Reserve 1 salmon filet for tomorrow's lunch.

2. Rinse lentils and cover with plenty of water. Bring to boil, reduce heat to low, and simmer for 20 minutes until tender, then drain. Sauté shallots in canola oil until lightly browned. Stir in the salt and the remaining ingredients into the drained lentils and serve with salmon.

2B: Grilled Salmon Salad

Serves 1

1 cooked filet of salmon

2-3 cups mixed greens

2 tablespoons sliced green onions

2 tablespoons sliced almonds

2 tablespoons garbanzo beans

2 tablespoons fresh berries

2 tablespoons Lemon-thyme Vinaigrette (recipe towards end of chapter)

Toss all ingredients together and drizzle dressing over salad.

3A: Pan-seared Pork with White Beans
Serves 2-3

1 pork tenderloin (approximately 1 pound) cut into 1" slices (or 3 boneless pork chops)

1 teaspoon all-purpose seasoning blend (recipe towards end of chapter)

1 tablespoon canola oil

1 large sliced onion

1 clove chopped garlic

2 teaspoons chopped fresh sage

1 can (15-oz.) white beans, drained and rinsed

½ cup white wine

1. Season the pork and pan sear with onions on medium high heat for 2-4 minutes on each side until browned. Remove pork from pan and set aside and cover. Reserve some pork for tomorrow's lunch.
2. Add remaining ingredients to pan with onions and cook on medium low heat until heated throughout. Serve the pork over beans.

3B: Pork and Lentil Salad

Serves 1

Sliced cooked pork
1 ½ cups chopped fresh vegetables such as broccoli, cucumber, mushrooms
½ cup dry lentils
½ cup diced tomato
2 tablespoons diced red bell pepper
2 tablespoons Balsamic Vinaigrette (recipe towards end of chapter)
¼ teaspoon salt

1. Rinse lentils and cover with plenty of water. Bring to boil, reduce heat to low and simmer for 20 minutes until tender, then drain.
2. Stir together all ingredients. Chill overnight.

4A: Southwestern Chicken and Quinoa

Serves 2-3

3 chicken breast halves, about the size of a deck of cards
1 teaspoon all-purpose seasoning blend (recipe towards end of chapter)
1 teaspoon chili powder
½ teaspoon cumin
1 tablespoon canola oil
1 ½ cup dry quinoa
1 can (10-oz.) of chopped tomatoes with chiles

1 cup water
½ cup shredded cheddar cheese

1. Bring quinoa, water, and canned tomatoes with juice to boil, stir, cover, and reduce heat to low. Simmer for 15-20 minutes. Let set for 5 minutes, uncovered, off the heat, then fluff with a fork.
2. If the chicken breast is thick, slice into two pieces horizontally. Season all breasts with all-purpose seasoning. Season 2 breasts with remaining spices. Grill or broil all chicken breasts on medium high heat for 10-12 minutes until cooked through. Reserve the breast with only all-purpose seasoning for tomorrow's lunch.
3. Slice chicken and serve over quinoa. Top with cheddar cheese.

4B: Orchard Spinach Salad
Serves 1

2-3 cups spinach
1 cooked sliced chicken breast
½ pear sliced
2 tablespoons chopped pecans
2 tablespoons sliced green onion
2 tablespoons Lemon-thyme Vinaigrette (recipe towards end of chapter)

Toss all ingredients together and drizzle dressing over salad.

5A: Chicken Stir-fry

Serves 2-3

3 chicken breast halves, sliced into thin strips
1 tablespoon canola oil
1 teaspoon all-purpose seasoning blend (recipe towards end of chapter)
1 clove chopped garlic
1 teaspoon chopped fresh ginger
1 cup finely chopped broccoli
¼ cup diced red bell peppers
2 tablespoons sliced green onions
1 tablespoon lime juice
1 tablespoon soy sauce
¾ cup bulgur wheat
1 ½ cups water

1. Combine chicken, oil, spices, and garlic and marinate overnight. Sauté on high heat for 6-8 minutes until cooked through. Remove chicken to a plate and cover. Reserve a portion of chicken for tomorrow's lunch.
2. Add vegetables, ginger, and canola oil to skillet and sauté quickly for 3-4 minutes.
3. Bring bulgur and water to boil, reduce heat to low and simmer for 15-20 minutes. Serve with sautéed chicken and vegetables on top of bulgur. Drizzle with soy sauce and lime juice and top with green onions.

5B: *Mediterranean Chicken Salad*
Serves 1

1 portion cooked sliced chicken breast
1 cup drained and rinsed red beans
2 tablespoons sliced frozen or canned artichokes (rinsed well)
2 tablespoons diced onion
½ cup chopped fresh broccoli
¼ cup diced cucumber
½ cup diced tomato
2 tablespoons crumbled feta cheese
2 tablespoons Balsamic Vinaigrette (recipe towards end of chapter)

Stir together all ingredients. Chill overnight.

6A: *Herbed Bulgur-stuffed Chicken*
Serves 2-3

3 chicken breast halves, each about the size of a deck of cards
1 cup dry bulgur
2 cups water
2 tablespoons diced red bell peppers
2 tablespoons onion, diced
3 sprigs of fresh thyme
½ teaspoon chopped fresh sage
1 clove chopped garlic
1 tablespoon lemon juice

1 tablespoon olive oil

2 teaspoons all-purpose seasoning blend (recipe towards end of chapter)

½ teaspoon salt

1. Bring bulgur and water to boil, reduce heat to low and simmer for 15-20 minutes. Reserve ½ cup for tomorrow's lunch.
2. Combine cooked bulgur, diced vegetables, herbs, garlic, lemon, and oil for stuffing. Add salt and mix.
3. Cut a pocket in 2 chicken breasts with a knife. Stuff each pocket with the bulgur mixture. Season all chicken breasts and bake at 375 on greased baking sheet for 25-30 minutes until cooked through. Reserve unstuffed chicken breast for tomorrow's lunch.

6B: Bulgur Chicken Salad

Serves 1

½ cup cooked bulgur

1 cooked diced chicken breast

2 tablespoons diced red onion

2 tablespoons red bell pepper, diced

1 cup additional vegetables such as sliced Brussels sprouts, asparagus, or kale

2 tablespoons Lemon-thyme Vinaigrette (recipe towards end of chapter)

2 tablespoons chopped walnuts

1 tablespoon parmesan cheese
1 tablespoon chopped dried cranberries

Stir together all ingredients. Chill overnight.

7A: Roasted Garlic Chicken with Creamy Mashed Cauliflower
Serves 2-3

3 chicken breast halves, about the size of a deck of cards
1 ½ teaspoon all-purpose seasoning blend (recipe towards end
of chapter)
1 tablespoon olive oil
2 tablespoons roasted garlic
3 cups finely chopped cauliflower
2 tablespoons water
3 sprigs fresh thyme
½ cup plain or Greek strained yogurt
1 teaspoon salt

1. Combine seasoning blend, roasted garlic, and oil; use to
   marinate the chicken overnight.
2. Place cauliflower in a microwave-safe bowl with water;
   cover and steam in a microwave oven on high setting for
   3 to 5 minutes, until very tender.
3. Bake chicken breasts on greased baking sheet at 375 for
   20 minutes. Reserve 1 breast for tomorrow's lunch.
4. Combine cooked cauliflower and remaining ingredients
   in food processor; add the salt and blend until smooth.
   Top with sliced chicken breasts.

7B: Black Bean Chicken Salad
Serves 1

1 baked and diced garlic chicken breast
1 cup drained and rinsed black beans
2 tablespoons diced red onion
2 tablespoons diced red bell pepper
2 tablespoons diced tomato
1 ½ cups chopped fresh vegetables such as broccoli, cucumber, or cauliflower
2 tablespoons Cilantro Vinaigrette (recipe towards end of chapter)

Stir together all ingredients. Chill overnight.

8A: Grilled Flank Steak
Serves 2-3

1 flank or skirt steak
2 tablespoons olive oil
4 cloves chopped garlic
Zest and juice of 1 lime (see notes on zesting towards end of chapter)
¼ cup chopped fresh cilantro
1 sliced large red bell pepper
1 sliced large onion
1 tablespoon canola oil

2 sprouted grain or whole grain pita breads

1. Combine olive oil, garlic, lime, and cilantro and marinate the beef overnight. Grill on medium high heat for 3-6 minutes per side to your preferred level of doneness. Note: Both these cuts of beef are most tender if served medium rare. Let the beef rest for 5 minutes before slicing thin against the grain. Reserve some sliced beef for tomorrow's lunch.

2. Sauté onions and peppers in canola oil for 4-6 minutes on high heat. Serve with sliced beef inside toasted pita bread.

8B: Steak and Black Bean Salad

Serves 1

Cooked flank or skirt steak
1 cup drained and rinsed black beans
2 tablespoons diced red onion
2 tablespoons diced red bell pepper
2 tablespoons diced tomato
1 ½ cups chopped fresh vegetables such as broccoli, cucumber, or mushrooms
2 tablespoons Cilantro Vinaigrette (recipe towards end of chapter)

Stir together all ingredients. Chill overnight.

9A: Lemon Artichoke Grilled Shrimp
Serves 2-3

1 ½ pound peeled and de-veined shrimp
4 tablespoons Lemon-thyme Vinaigrette (recipe towards end of chapter)
1 clove garlic, chopped
1 cup dry quinoa
2 cups water
2 tablespoons parmesan cheese
½ cup frozen or canned artichokes, rinsed and sliced

1. Combine shrimp, vinaigrette, and garlic and marinate overnight.
2. Bring quinoa and water to boil, stir, cover, and reduce heat to low and simmer for 15-20 minutes. Let sit for 5 minutes, uncovered, off heat, then stir in the artichokes. Note: you may also use a rice cooker to prepare the quinoa, using the same proportion of water.
3. Grill shrimp on medium heat for 6-8 minutes or sauté for 6-8 minutes on medium high heat. Reserve some shrimp for tomorrow's lunch. Serve shrimp atop quinoa with parmesan cheese.

9B: Greek Shrimp Salad
Serves 1

Marinated cooked lemon shrimp
2-3 cups mixed greens

¼ diced red bell pepper

½ cup frozen or canned artichokes, rinsed and sliced

2 tablespoons feta cheese

2 tablespoons red wine vinegar for dressing

Toss all ingredients together and drizzle dressing over salad.

10A: Pan-fried Teriyaki Tofu and Rice
Serves 2-3

1 package extra firm tofu

¼ cup low-sodium soy sauce

2 cloves chopped garlic

1 teaspoon chopped fresh ginger

2 teaspoons sherry or rice wine vinegar

1 teaspoon honey

¾ cup black (or brown) rice

1 ½ cups water

¼ cup diced sweet red bell pepper

¼ cup diced onion

1 tablespoon canola oil

¼ cup chopped broccoli

¼ cup fresh asparagus cut into 1" sections

1 tablespoon soy sauce

1. Drain tofu and slice into ½" thick sticks. Lay tofu between paper towels and press firmly to extract as much liquid as possible.

2. Combine soy, garlic, ginger, sherry, and honey and marinate tofu for one hour.

3. Bring rice and water to boil, reduce heat to low, and cover to simmer for 15-20 minutes or until rice is cooked through. Or, use a rice cooker with the same proportion of water.

4. Remove tofu from marinade and pat dry. Pan fry in skillet with a small amount of oil on medium low heat until golden brown and crispy on all sides. Reserve some of the cooked tofu for tomorrow's lunch.

5. Sauté onion and pepper in canola oil for 4-6 minutes until nicely browned and translucent. Stir in the remaining vegetables and cook for an additional 4-6 minutes until tender. Stir vegetables into cooked rice and top with tofu.

10B: Teriyaki Tofu Salad
Serves 1

2-3 cups mixed greens
Marinated and pan-fried tofu
¼ cup chopped fresh broccoli
¼ cup fresh sugar snap peas
2 tablespoons diced red bell pepper
1 tablespoon sliced green onions
1 tablespoon sliced almonds
2 tablespoons Sesame Vinaigrette (recipe towards chapter end)

Toss all ingredients together and drizzle dressing over salad.

Zesting

To zest a lemon, lime, or orange, scrape it gently on a fine grater and collect the shavings. Avoid getting into the white layer of pith underneath.

Vinaigrettes
Lemon-thyme Vinaigrette

¼ cup olive oil

Zest and juice of 1 lemon (see previous notes on zesting)

3 sprigs fresh thyme

Pinch of salt

Pinch of cracked pepper

1 teaspoon chopped fresh sage

Store in a jar with a tightly fitting lid. The vinaigrette will keep in the refrigerator up to a week. Shake well before using.

Balsamic Vinaigrette

¼ cup balsamic vinegar

¼ cup olive oil

1 teaspoon Italian Seasoning Blend

1 clove minced garlic

1 pinch of salt

1/8 teaspoon cracked black pepper

Store in a jar with a tightly fitting lid. The vinaigrette will keep in the refrigerator up to a week. Shake well before using.

Cilantro Vinaigrette
Zest and juice of 1 lime (see previous notes on zesting)
2 cloves minced garlic
¼ cup apple cider vinegar
2/3 cup cilantro leaves
¼ cup olive oil
Pinch of salt
Pinch of cracked pepper

Store in a jar with a tightly fitting lid. The vinaigrette will keep in the refrigerator up to a week. Shake well before using.

Sesame Vinaigrette
2 tablespoons sesame oil
2 tablespoons olive oil
¼ cup apple cider vinegar
1 clove minced garlic
½ teaspoon fresh ginger

Store in a jar with a tightly fitting lid. The vinaigrette will keep in the refrigerator up to a week. Shake well before using.

All-purpose seasoning blend
1 tablespoon onion powder
1 tablespoon garlic powder
1 teaspoon sea salt
½ teaspoon black pepper
½ teaspoon paprika

Chapter 39

Salads

A salad is an excellent tune-up meal. While salads are traditionally associated with leaves, there is no rule that says a salad has to have leaves. Non-leafy vegetables, fruits, beans, and meats provide an almost infinite variety to salads, and there are always new taste combinations to be discovered. Keep experimenting, and you will never be bored of eating salads.

If you have little or no experience in salad-making, below are some suggestions you might find helpful. Pick one or more ingredients from each section and chop as necessary. Transfer to a bowl, add the dressing, and mix. If you are not going to eat the whole amount right away, add dressing only to what you will eat now and refrigerate the rest.

If you are tired of eating leaves—this is a common complaint—use only a small amount of leaves or none at all.

Leaves

Such as red leaf lettuce, romaine lettuce, iceberg lettuce, arugula, spinach, micro-greens, and herbs.

Fresh leaves taste better than the bagged variety, but the bagged ones are easier to use. Fresh leaves should be washed thoroughly under running water or in a bowl that has water running continuously through it, and then dried with paper towels or in a spinner. Bagged leaves that do not say "pre-washed" or "ready to eat" should also be washed.

Vegetables

Such as mushrooms, tomatoes, cucumbers, radishes, bell peppers, jicama root, green onion, carrots, broccoli, and cauliflower.

Beans

Such as garbanzo, pinto, black, red, cannelloni, and also bean sprouts.

Fruits

Such as apples, pears, grapes (in moderation), strawberries, oranges (fresh mandarin orange sections are great), olives, and pomegranates.

Cheese

Such as shredded or cubed cheddar, Swiss, parmesan, crumbled feta, sliced mozzarella.

Meat/Eggs

Such as baked, broiled, or grilled chicken; grilled, baked, or poached salmon; canned light tuna (in moderation); sliced steak; deli meats (in moderation); sliced boiled eggs (but not if you had an egg for breakfast).

Dressings

A combination of

    a) red wine, rice wine, or balsamic vinegar along with

    b) fresh lemon, lime, or orange juice,

    c) olive oil, and

    d) a pinch of salt

makes for a quick and surprisingly tasty dressing. Play around with the amount of each ingredient to suit your taste.

You may have already tried the vinaigrettes in chapter 21. If you are ready for something more ambitious, check out the vinaigrette recipes in chapter 38.

When using a creamy dressing, don't pour the dressing over your salad. Keep the dressing separate (on the side) and dip your fork in it before spearing each bite. You will use less dressing and the salad will taste just as good.

Kitchen Tools

Consider purchasing the following: an apple corer, vegetable peeler, egg slicer, cheese grater and a paring knife. While not essential, these do make salad preparation go a little faster.

Preparing a tasty, visually appealing salad takes a few minutes, but it's worth the effort. Eating a salad is eating as close to nature as you can get. Think about this—each time you make and eat a salad, you have taken another step towards better health. You are giving yourself the opportunity to live the life you've dreamed of living.

Made in the USA
Lexington, KY
17 July 2014